The Maudsley

ANTIPSYCHOTIC

MEDICATION REVIEW

SERVICE GUIDELINES

Ruth Ohlsen RGN RMN Dip Nut
Clinical Research Nurse
Institute of Psychiatry
London, UK

Shubulade Smith MBBS MRCPsych FRSM
Consultant Psychiatrist, Maudsley Hospital
South London and Maudsley NHS Trust
London, UK

David Taylor BSc MSc MRPharmS
Chief Pharmacist, South London and Maudsley NHS Trust
and Honorary Senior Lecturer, Institute of Psychiatry
London, UK

Lyn Pilowsky BM BS MRCPsych PhD
Reader in Neurochemical Imaging and Psychiatry
Medical Research Council Senior Clinical Fellow
Honorary Consultant Psychiatrist
South London and Maudsley NHS Trust
London, UK

MARTIN DUNITZ

First published in the United Kingdom in 2003
by Martin Dunitz, an imprint of the Taylor & Francis Group plc, 11 New Fetter Lane, London EC4P 4EE

Tel.: +44 (0) 20 7583 9855
Fax.: +44 (0) 20 7842 2298
E-mail: info@dunitz.co.uk
Website: http://www.dunitz.co.uk

Reprinted 2004

Although every effort has been made to ensure that drug doses and other information are presented accurately in this publication, the ultimate responsibility rests with the prescribing physician. Neither the publishers nor the authors can be held responsible for errors or for any consequences arising from the use of information contained herein. For detailed prescribing information or instructions on the use of any product or procedure discussed herein, please consult the prescribing information or instructional material issued by the manufacturer.

A CIP record for this book is available from the British Library.

ISBN 1-84184-221-4

Distributed in the USA by
Fulfilment Center
Taylor & Francis
10650 Toebben Drive
Independence, KY 41051, USA
Toll Free Tel.: +1 800 634 7064
E-mail: taylorandfrancis@thomsonlearning.com

Distributed in Canada by
Taylor & Francis
74 Rolark Drive
Scarborough, Ontario M1R 4G2, Canada
Toll Free Tel.: +1 877 226 2237
E-mail: tal_fran@istar.ca

Distributed in the rest of the world by
Thomson Publishing Services
Cheriton House
North Way
Andover, Hampshire SP10 5BE, UK
Tel.: +44 (0)1264 332424
E-mail: salesorder.tandf@thomsonpublishingservices.co.uk

Composition by Wearset Ltd, Boldon, Tyne and Wear.
Printed and bound in Great Britain by The Cromwell Press Ltd

Authors and editors

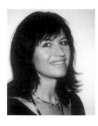

Ruth Ohlsen
Ruth Ohlsen has trained as a general and psychiatric nurse and has had many years experience in acute adult psychiatry. She managed the Maudsley Hospital clozapine clinic for over five years and was instrumental in setting up the Maudsley Atypical Antipsychotic Clinic (later the Maudsley Medication Review Clinic). She has extensive experience in medication and side-effect management, and has managed the Atypical Clinic Dietary Advice Service for the last two years. She has acted as Nursing Team Manager for the Southwark First Onset Psychosis Team (FIRST) since January 2001, and is doing a PhD and associated research projects on the mechanisms and management of antipsychotic induced weight gain.

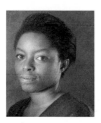

Shubulade Smith
Shubulade Smith is a consultant psychiatrist at the North East Lambeth sector of the South London and Maudsley NHS Trust. She runs a community team serving the Brixton area and ES3, an acute adult ward at the Maudsley Hospital. In addition, she is attached to the Department of Psychological Medicine at the Institute of Psychiatry. Dr Smith runs a research group investigating the effects of antipsychotics on bone and physical health. Prior to this, Dr Smith worked with Dr Lyn Pilowsky at the Maudsley Atypical Antipsychotic Clinic and initiated a medication review service at her community mental health team base.

Dr Smith completed a clinical research fellowship examining the endocrine side effects of antipsychotic medication, supervised by Professor Robin Murray at the Institute of Psychiatry.

Her research has shown that older antipsychotic medications do have profound and lasting effects on sexual and reproductive function. Having found significant proportions of people suffering with physical problems, Dr Smith is now setting up a joint medication review/GP outreach clinic at the team base, a 'one-stop shop' aimed at health promotion and management of physical problems in people with severe mental illness.

Dr Smith trained in medicine at Guy's Hospital, London before training in postgraduate psychiatry at the Maudsley Hospital.

Dr Smith was nominated as one of the 'Women of the Year 2002' for trying to improve services for patients with severe mental illness.

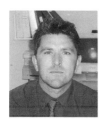

David Taylor
David Taylor is Chief Pharmacist at the South London and Maudsley NHS Trust, Honorary Senior Lecturer at the Institute of Psychiatry and Foundation President of the College of Mental Health Pharmacists. His main areas of research are pharmacokinetics and prescribing practice in mental health. His team at the Maudsley is widely involved in systemic reviews and meta-analyses of psychotropic drug therapy. David is lead author of the *Maudsley 2001 Prescribing Guidelines* (Martin Dunitz, 2001) and co-editor of *Case Studies in Psychopharmacology* (Martin Dunitz, 1998).

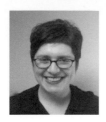

Lyn Pilowsksy
In 1986, on completion of her medical training in Australia, Lyn Pilowsky came to the Maudsley Hospital to specialise in psychiatry. During her specialist training she performed a survey of rapid tranquillisation (the largest naturalistic survey of emergency drug administration in the literature). Lyn came to work with Professor Robin Murray's schizrenia group in 1990 at the Institute of Psychiatry, and helped collect multiple affected families for genetic linkage and association studies.

At this time, Lyn was awarded a Wellcome Trust Junior Research Fellowship to work with Professors Rob Kerwin (IOP) and Peter Ell (Institute of Nuclear Medicine (IONM), Middlesex Hospital, London) and began a programme of studies using in vivo receptor measurement with single photon emission tomography (SPET), to evaluate the dopamine hypothesis of schizophrenia in living human subjects. This work results in a PhD in 1994. A Medical Research Council (MRC) Clinician Scientist Award allowed consolidation of this initial effort. Dr Pilowsky was at the hub of a team investigating limbic dopamine D2 receptors, 5HT2a and GABA receptors in schizophrenia, alcohol dependence and depression and, through this work, was granted the title of Reader in Neurochemical Imaging, London University. With further generous support in the form of an MRC Senior Clinical Research Fellowship in 1999, Dr Pilowsky now leads a team at the IONM and IOP studying systems involved in presynaptic control of dopamine including NMDA and sigma receptors and heads the Section of Neurochemical Imaging and Psychiatry at the IOP and with charitable industrial sponsorship from AstraZeneca, Novartis, Janssen and Synthelabo, has expanded her team's research portfolio to include research projects into antipsychotic induced weight gain, fMRI studies of cortical function in first episode schizophrenia, and the neuropsychology of negative symptoms. Dr Pilowsky encourages and supports junior researchers training in this field and has led clinical teams as Consultant Psychiatrist to the Maudsley Psychiatric Intensive Care Unit, and the Maudsley Antipsychotic Medication Review Service. With a charitable award from AstraZeneca, Dr Pilowsky developed and now leads a new service, the Southwark First Onset Psychosis Service (FIRST) aimed at systematic and close care of patients in their first episode of psychosis, which allow her to pursue her interests in the management of the severely mentally ill, and the neuropharmacology of psychosis.

Contents

Disclaimer

The opinions expressed are those of the individual authors in consultation with various international experts and with the South London and Maudsley NHS Trust's Drug and Therapeutics Committee. Every care has been taken to ensure that these Guidelines are up-to-date and accurate. However, it must be considered that this document is but the end product of reasoned influences from several clinicians. We do not claim that every piece of advice provided is 'correct', only that we have taken care to ensure that advice is based on firm evidence and clinical experience. We hope to have included all information available to us in July 2002, but this will inevitably become out-dated as time goes by. Readers should bear this in mind and should always consult the latest manufacturers' information and the British National Formulary or the equivalent text for their country of practice.

It is also important to recognise that Clinical Practice differs from one country to another and that availability and licensing of drugs discussed in these Guidelines also vary with geographical location. Please note that many of the drugs listed in the tables are done so alphabetically and not necessarily in order of preference. Generic drugs may require special care and attention in relation to dosage and use. Special attention should always be paid to contraindications and side effects. Many of the drugs discussed are not yet available in some countries and many of the uses may be 'off licence' in the UK as well as overseas. Similarly, recommended doses vary greatly from country to country. The normal serum and plasma levels quoted may vary from country to country, and between individual laboratories in the UK. Clinicians are strongly advised to check their local laws and local hospital or national clinical guidelines before using any information in a clinical situation. The clinical care of any individual patient remains at all times that of the treating psychiatrist or other clinician. Additional terms and conditions may apply and may be notified. All regulatory bodies will be those of the United Kingdom and the law of England will apply in all matters relating to the *Maudsley Antipsychotic Medication Review Guidelines*. No liability is accepted for any injury, loss or damage howsoever caused.

Foreword

Antipsychotic drugs have been the mainstay of treatment for schizophrenia since their introduction in the 1950s. Over the following 30 years, no clear differences emerged between the available agents in their therapeutic efficacy or clinical predictors of response. Thus, a clinician's choice of drug for an acute psychotic episode or long-term relapse prevention was based primarily on factors such as perceived side-effect profile and whether a depot preparation was available. Antipsychotics were seen as essentially safe drugs whose dosage could be raised with relative impunity, higher dosage being the most common therapeutic strategy for an unresponsive illness. When weighing up the risks against the benefits, the primary consideration was the common occurrence of extrapyramidal side-effects. Initially, the focus was on acute movement disorder such as parkinsonism, akathisia and dystonia, but in the 1970s there was increased awareness of later-onset, long-term problems such as tardive dyskinesia.

In the late 1980s, the drug clozapine was revived. Thorough re-assessment established that this had a superior efficacy for schizophrenia that was otherwise unresponsive to antipsychotics as well as a lower liability for movement disorders. While the drug carried the risk of potentially fatal agranulocytosis and other serious side-effects, its efficacy in treatment-resistant schizophrenia and the emerging claims for superior benefit for negative symptoms and cognitive deficits led to careful review of the risk–benefit balance for treatment strategies in people whose schizophrenia had proved refractory to medication. The 1990s saw the introduction of a range of other so-called atypical or second-generation antipsychotics, which shared some of the advantages of clozapine, particularly the reduced likelihood of inducing movement disorder, but varied in their propensity to cause a range of other side-effects, such as weight gain, diabetes and cardiovascular effects. For some of these agents, study findings suggested some benefits in patients with a poor response to conventional antipsychotic medication. However, the evidence for efficacy in strictly defined, treatment-resistant schizophrenia only remained convincing for clozapine.

The widespread clinical use of clozapine and the other newer antipsychotics, and the experience of improved tolerability and better efficacy, raised expectations among clinicians and those receiving such medication. This stimulated an increased readiness to adjust dosage, switch medication and consider adjunctive strategies in order to obtain the optimum response and minimise side-effects. However, the evidence base relevant to the regular review of antipsychotic drug regimens and consideration of further interventions was growing rapidly, with fresh evidence continually emerging on the relative risks and benefits of each of the second-generation antipsychotics.

It was in this context that the antipsychotic medication review service at the Maudsley Hospital was established. The authors of this book have brought together their expertise and experience of working in that service, carefully treating and monitoring patients referred because of intolerance of, or poor response to, conventional antipsychotic medication. In an early chapter they review the pharmacology of the antipsychotic drugs and the mechanisms relevant to therapeutic efficacy and side-effects. Next, they examine the evidence base of systematic review and meta-analyses of clinical trial data, particularly in respect of key clinical questions regarding the efficacy, tolerability and safety of the newer drugs. This is followed by the key section of the book, which describes the principles and procedures of the antipsychotic medication review service. For example, emphasis is placed on the importance of obtaining a comprehensive medication history, gathering information on whether adequate trials of past treatments were administered, and the nature and extent of the therapeutic response, side-effects and concordance. The authors provide details of their methods of assessment, including the use of formal rating scales, and demonstrate how these may be incorporated into clinical practice, as part of the regular review of patients by community mental health teams. They also provide information on common drug interactions and side-effects, and practical advice on managing switches of medication. A series of convincing case reports illustrate how the principles of medication management may be applied in clinical practice.

In short, this book sets out the basis for the rational prescribing of antipsychotic medication. For those of us involved in the use of these drugs in adult mental health, it reminds us of what we know, what we think we know (although careful analysis of the evidence base may reveal considerable uncertainty), and what we do not know. And it also shows us what we should be doing.

Thomas Barnes
Imperial College Faculty of Medicine, London

Preface

Since the introduction of antipsychotic prescribing in the early 1950s, clinical practice in psychiatry has changed almost beyond recognition. The variety of antipsychotic drugs now available presents clinicians today with an abundance of choice that, while welcome, can in reality be quite bewildering. The prevention and management of treatment-emergent side-effects, and the evaluation of antipsychotic treatment is an ongoing process, requiring time, knowledge and systematic review, and it was to this end that the Maudsley Medication Review Service was initiated.

This is not a guide to first-line prescribing, but is intended for use in conjunction with the *Maudsley Prescribing Guidelines*. The purpose of the *Maudsley Antipsychotic Medication Review Service Guidelines* is to give straightforward information and practical advice about managing aspects of ongoing antipsychotic treatment. We have found a systematic and holistic approach to patient care to be beneficial, and hope that the book will be of practical help to clinicians wishing to set up their own Medication Review Clinics. The advice given herein is based on our own clinical experience, on the current literature and on expert opinions provided by other clinicians. The book is written from a variety of professional backgrounds, each author bringing their individual fields of expertise and clinical experience. We believe the *Maudsley Antipsychotic Medication Review Service Guidelines* will be accessible and useful to almost anybody involved in caring for people with serious mental illness.

Ruth Ohlsen
October 2002

1 The Maudsley Medication Review Service – an evolving strategy

The 1990s heralded a revolution in the pharmacological management of schizophrenia. The re-emergence of clozapine, and evidence for its efficacy even in treatment-resistant patient groups, stimulated antipsychotic drug discovery. Many new compounds were brought to therapeutic use.

The Maudsley Antipsychotic Medication Review Service was developed primarily as a 'test-bed' for atypical antipsychotic drugs so that a level of expertise with these compounds could build up and inform practice throughout the trust. Before that, information on new atypical antipsychotic drugs in naturalistic settings was anecdotal and sparse. The goal of the service was to give patients, intolerant or poorly responsive to typical antipsychotic medication, a chance to try novel atypical antipsychotic drugs in a systematic fashion, and to be monitored and closely supervised by senior psychiatric and nursing staff. The Maudsley Medication Review Service was conceived as both a centre of, and a place to develop expertise with patients in an evidence-based fashion. The intention was also to try to adhere to clinical standards which would form part of an audit cycle. These standards were:

+ To avoid extrapyramidal side-effects
+ To avoid hyperprolactinaemia
+ To avoid antipsychotic polypharmacy
+ To avoid anticholinergic medication
+ To avoid weight gain
+ To systematically evaluate progress with formal clinical rating scales.

Patients were followed for 2 years and the service was independently audited (Stone et al, 2002). Data revealed that patients improved symptomatically and functionally. It was found to be possible to switch the majority of patients from typical antipsychotic treatment to atypical antipsychotic monotherapy without adverse consequences.

As the service evolved, referrals came from standard care settings asking simply for a thorough review of their patients' medication in the light of their past history and present state. In many cases the review was driven by user dissatisfaction with side-effects, or a wish by the referrer to get another opinion. The medication review became an opportunity where patient and carers could gather information and engage in a dialogue about the options available. Often the decision was taken to stay on the same regimen.

The opinion of the Medication Review Service and clinical ratings of the patient were made available to the consulting referrer and acted as a benchmark for future care. It became obvious that this was a model of care that could be transferred to standard clinics. Instead of attendance at a depot clinic for passive receipt of medication (which might nevertheless be entirely appropriate), these clinics could be modernized to act as centres for a therapeutic revamp, even in chronic, apparently stabilized patients. The Medication Review Service would provide a critical reassessment normally only available to patients at times of (unwished for) crisis – for example, ward summaries obtained after an inpatient admission. Here we have attempted to distil the principles and practice of an approach that can be incorporated into standard care settings, and provide a general approach for evidence-based antipsychotic prescribing.

2 The pharmacology of atypical antipsychotic drugs

The primary distinction between typical and atypical antipsychotic drugs is clinical, rather than mechanistic. Atypical antipsychotic drugs have a wide risk:benefit ratio, and have a diminished or absent tendency to induce extrapyramidal side-effects at therapeutically useful doses. Although it is not clearly understood why this may be so, neuropharmacological studies support biological distinctions between typical and atypical antipsychotic drugs and these are briefly reviewed below.

Animal behavioural studies

Inhibition of a conditioned avoidance response has been widely used as an animal test predictive of the antipsychotic potential of a compound, while induction of catalepsy in rats is associated with the occurrence of extrapyramidal side-effects (EPS) in the clinic (Moore et al, 1993). The atypical antipsychotic drugs olanzapine, risperidone, clozapine and ziprasidone (Seeger et al, 1995) show greater 'separation' of these effects than the reference typical antipsychotic haloperidol. The implication of these screening tests is that compounds with 'atypical' properties will have a wide therapeutic ratio between antipsychotic and extrapyramidal effects. The therapeutic window may still vary between drugs, but is greater than for the typical agents. Importantly, these tests do not imply particular mechanisms for atypicality, and different drugs may arrive at this profile by differing mechanisms (Kerwin, 1994).

Electrophysiology data

These data relate to the effect of antipsychotic drugs on depolarization of dopamine neurons in the substantia nigra (SN) (nigro-striatal pathways) and the ventral tegmental area (VTA) (mesolimbic and mesocortical areas), to evaluate the likelihood that a drug will induce extrapyramidal side-effects (EPS). Drugs that are less likely to cause EPS have a more selective effect on the VTA. Direct injections of muscimol into the VTA and SN have been used to selectively stimulate the mesolimbic and striato-nigral pathways, respectively. In one study, haloperidol and fluphenazine inhibited stimulation of both pathways, whereas the relatively lower potency (meaning a lower affinity for blocking dopamine D2 receptors) antipsychotic drugs thioridazine and clozapine inhibited stimulation of the VTA responses more potently (Oakley et al, 1991). Interestingly, it appears that selective effects on mesolimbic pathways are related to duration of exposure to the drug. Clozapine increases the firing rate of both nigro-striatal and mesolimbic dopaminergic neurons after acute administration, but only the mesolimbic population exhibits chronic depolarization blockade after repeated exposure to the drug. Classic antipsychotic treatment results in depolarization blockade of both groups of neurons after chronic treatment (Coward et al, 1989).

Receptor binding in vitro

Meltzer and Matsubara (1989) examined potential receptor binding characteristics that could account for a profile of clinical efficacy and low extrapyramidal side-effects. They showed that the

5HT2a/D2 ratio was most successful at classifying antipsychotic drugs. Drugs with greater action at 5HT2a than at D2 receptors were more likely to have therapeutic efficacy with few or no EPS. The serotonergic system regulates dopamine transmission in striatal regions and antagonism of 5HT2a receptors was thought to offset the risk of EPS caused by dopamine D2 blockade. There is still incomplete agreement as to the in vitro receptor profile, which will, with certainty, produce therapeutic benefit without motor side-effects. Some atypical drugs show a broad spectrum of action at many receptor sites, with modest or very modest potency at blocking D2 receptors (clozapine and quetiapine), whilst other broad spectrum drugs show high potency at both 5HT2a and D2 receptors (risperidone, olanzapine and ziprasidone) (Seeger et al, 1995), and others (amisulpride) have negligible action for any receptor site apart from dopamine receptor subtypes (D2 and D3 receptors). It appears that there are a range of mechanisms by which a drug can be atypical, but certainly the drugs which show placebo level EPS and prolactin level elevation across a range of doses (i.e. the most robustly 'atypical') have a broad yet modest spectrum of action across a wide range of receptor targets (clozapine and quetiapine).

It is clear that precise neuroreceptor targets, which are beneficial without adverse effects, are yet to be identified. Many targets (e.g. glutamate, serotonergic and sigma), are awaiting technical developments in order to progress the field. Lidow et al (1998) have shown in primates that chronic treatment with the atypical antipsychotic drugs clozapine and olanzapine selectively upregulates cortical dopamine D2/D3 receptors, but is without effect in the striatum. This was not the case for the typical antipsychotic drug haloperidol, which upregulated dopamine D2/D3 receptor binding nonselectively in both striatum and cortex. A selective action at limbic cortical dopamine receptors could also account for an atypical profile of antipsychotic efficacy without motor side-effects.

Effects on cellular mechanisms in the brain

After depolarization, the neuron responds by expressing genes to manufacture intracellular proteins needed for signalling pathways. One such 'early gene family' (*fos*) measurably increases in concentration as a consequence of synaptic activation (Robertson and Fibiger, 1991). This has led to the proposal that *fos* immunohistochemistry may be used to map functional response pathways in the CNS.

When administered to rats, haloperidol and raclopride both produced large increases in the number of c-*fos*-containing neurons in the striatum and nucleus accumbens. Clozapine was without effect in the striatum but significantly induced the number of *fos*-positive neurons in the nucleus accumbens, medial prefrontal cortex, and lateral septal nucleus (limbic cortical neurons). This relative sparing of an effect on striatal neurons by clozapine has been supported by more recent work showing that chronic administration of haloperidol to rats dramatically induced delta*fos*B in the caudate putamen, with a smaller induction in the nucleus accumbens and prefrontal cortex. Clozapine failed to increase delta*fos*B in any of the three brain regions studied, and the atypical antipsychotic drugs risperidone and olanzapine produced significantly lower inductions in delta*fos*B in the caudate putamen than haloperidol, and similar effects to clozapine in the other brain regions (Atkins et al, 1999).

Implications of drug effects on cellular mechanisms

✦   Blockade of dopamine D2 receptors (at least) is a minimum requirement for a drug to have antipsychotic action.

◆ Dopamine D2 receptors are critical to pathways that regulate bodily movements and hormonal function, as well as mesocorticolimbic dopamine pathways, important to thinking, perception, emotion and behaviour (all of which are disrupted in schizophrenia).

◆ Biological evidence suggests that drugs likely to have an *atypical* clinical profile *selectively* act on mesolimbic and mesocortical dopamine pathways, and spare pathways associated with motor and hormonal function, where dopamine D2 receptor blockade produces undesirable motor (parkinsonian) and sexual side-effects.

Receptor binding in vivo: PET (positron emission tomography) and SPET (single photon emission tomography) studies in living subjects

In vivo studies of atypical antipsychotic drugs support the hypothesis that the ratio of 5HT2a:D2 receptor blockade is associated with their atypicality, and that typical antipsychotic drugs do not robustly express this characteristic. The atypical antipsychotic drugs clozapine, olanzapine, risperidone and quetiapine all share a high 5HT2a:D2 receptor occupancy profile in vivo (Gefvert et al, 1998; Travis et al, 1998; Kapur et al, 2000a). Typical antipsychotic drugs show either no occupancy of 5HT2a receptors in vivo (haloperidol), or modest occupancy rising with dose, and low 5HT2a:D2 occupancy ratios (chlorpromazine) (Trichard et al, 1998).

Clozapine and quetiapine show modest to low (or even transient) levels of striatal D2 receptor occupancy in vivo, and the blockade of these receptor sites is not dose dependent (Pilowsky et al, 1997; Kapur et al, 2000a; Stephenson et al, 2000). Risperidone and olanzapine both show dose-dependent occupancy of striatal D2 receptors, and risperidone has a somewhat narrower saturation curve than olanzapine (Kapur et al, 1999). Importantly, despite the fact that these drugs both exhibit nearly 100% occupancy of 5HT2a receptors, this does not protect against the appearance of EPS (suggesting that a high affinity for 5HT2a receptors may not in fact offset the risk of EPS-induced D2 receptor blockade, as was previously thought). Data on amisulpride, ziprasidone and zotepine are awaited, but it is likely from their in vivo receptor binding profile that they will show similar effects (dose-dependent occupancy) to risperidone and olanzapine at striatal D2 receptors. These observations are important, because Kapur et al (2000b) have shown that for haloperidol at least, the degree of striatal D2 occupancy relates to the onset of prolactin elevation and extrapyramidal side-effects (these effects occurring at around 72% and 78% striatal D2 receptor occupancy levels, respectively). Even doses of haloperidol as low as 2mg can induce striatal D2 occupancy values above 70% (Kapur et al, 1997). Studies of temporal cortical D2 receptors show that both typical and atypical antipsychotic drugs substantially block these receptors at clinically relevant doses, but that atypical antipsychotic drugs *preferentially* occupy these receptors, showing a higher 'limbic selective' D2 ratio than the typical antipsychotic drugs. Clozapine and quetiapine show this effect over a wide dose range (Pilowsky et al, 1997; Bigliani et al, 1999, 2000; Stephenson et al, 2000). Limbic cortical D2/D3 receptors are thought to be more relevant to the genesis of psychotic symptoms than striatal D2 receptor populations (Moore et al, 1999).

Summary

+ Data from in vivo receptor binding studies show that the atypical antipsychotic drugs clozapine, risperidone, olanzapine, and quetiapine all share strikingly high occupancy of cortical 5HT2a receptors.

+ Clinically relevant doses of these drugs (including amisulpride) attain preferential cortical vs striatal D2 occupancy levels (not true of typical antipsychotic drugs).

+ Animal data from behavioural, electrophysiology, *fos*-activation, and in vitro binding studies all support a mainly cortical site of action for atypical, compared with typical antipsychotic drugs.

+ These data are consistent with a high risk:benefit ratio (in relation both to EPS and hyperprolactinaemia) for these drugs.

3 The efficacy and tolerability of novel antipsychotic drugs

Recent reports on atypical antipsychotic drugs: The Cochrane Collaboration

The rigour, systematization, and full transparency of Cochrane reviews make them valuable resources. For this reason it is worth reporting the results of the main reviews of atypical antipsychotic drugs.

Clozapine vs typical antipsychotic drugs

Thirty one randomized controlled trials were reviewed comparing clozapine with typical antipsychotic drugs, of which 26 were <13 weeks in duration (Wahlbeck et al, 2000). The studies included 2589 participants. The authors reported no difference between the treatments with respect to mortality, ability to work, or time to discharge. There were, however, significant benefits in favour of clozapine in terms of clinical improvement and fewer relapses than with typical antipsychotic drugs. The clinical efficacy of clozapine was even more clearly superior to typical antipsychotic drugs in the treatment-resistant group in terms of clinical improvement and symptom reduction. Patients were more satisfied with clozapine treatment, and, longer term, found clozapine treatment more acceptable than conventional antipsychotic drugs. The side-effect profile of clozapine differed from that of conventional drugs. Patients on clozapine experienced hypersalivation, temperature increase, and drowsiness. Patients on conventional drugs experienced dry mouth and EPS effects. In their conclusions the authors comment that the short-term benefits of clozapine must be weighed against the risk of side-effects (in particular reduction in the white cell count). They confirm that clozapine is significantly more effective than typical antipsychotic drugs in producing meaningful clinical improvement, including postponing relapse. Nevertheless, they also state that the 'clinical effect of clozapine is at least in the short term not reflected in measures of global functioning, such as ability to leave hospital and maintain an occupation'. Conceding that this may be due to the short duration of the studies currently completed, they call for more community-based, long-term randomized trials to evaluate the efficacy of clozapine on global and social functioning in the community.

Olanzapine vs placebo and typical antipsychotic drugs

Randomized controlled trials comparing olanzapine with either placebo or typical antipsychotic drugs have been reviewed by Duggan et al (2000). The largest study included 1996 participants. Eight studies had <50 participants, five had 50 to 100 participants, and seven included more than 100 participants.

Olanzapine vs placebo

Over 300 citations were identified and nine trials were reviewed following literature searches. A further 11 randomized controlled trials were provided on application to Eli Lilly, bringing the total to 20 randomized controlled trials. The authors report a high patient attrition rate for olanzapine vs placebo comparisons over 6 weeks, although this favoured olanzapine (61% and 73% dropout from olanzapine and placebo, respectively). The authors urge caution in drawing firm conclusions from such trials with high dropout rates. Olanzapine-treated patients showed a significantly greater clinical response than placebo-treated individuals (defined as >40% reduction in psychotic symptoms). The effect was dose-related (greatest at 15mg, with declining effects at 10, 5, and 1mg). Olanzapine showed no particular advantage over placebo with respect to negative symptoms. Participants taking olanzapine were less likely to leave early due to lack of efficacy. Olanzapine patients showed placebo level need for anticholinergic and benzodiazepine medication. There were no clear differences between the groups in terms of EPS effects, and olanzapine in the doses used in these studies did not increase nausea and vomiting, sedation, agitation, hostility or withdrawal. Weight was increased after 6 weeks in the olanzapine-treated group but this was not statistically significant. At 6 months no clear difference in weight gain was shown between olanzapine and placebo. The reviewers noted that a range of important outcomes was not reported, including mortality, cognitive functioning, satisfaction with treatment, cost-effectiveness, social functioning and self-harm.

Olanzapine vs typical antipsychotic drugs

Eight randomized controlled trials were reviewed comparing olanzapine with haloperidol, four trials with chlorpromazine, and one trial each performed against perphenazine, fluphenazine, and flupenthixol. Data relating to 'no important clinical response' were not available in many of the papers reviewed. The available data favour olanzapine, but only if odds ratios, rather than relative risk data, are used (which is more conservative). One trial reported no difference between olanzapine and haloperidol in terms of relapse or readmission. The clinical global impression score was the same in the short term for patients treated with olanzapine and those treated with typical drugs, but a trend in favour of olanzapine appeared at the 3–12-month period. In terms of mental state, outcomes in the short and medium term favoured olanzapine. The negative symptoms subscale of the PANSS (Kay et al, 1987), BPRS (Overall and Gorham, 1962) and SANS (Andreasen, 1982) scales all favoured olanzapine in the short, medium and long term. For positive symptoms, PANSS-positive subscore rating was in favour of olanzapine, both in the short and the medium term. Data described by the reviewers as 'skewed' were reported as showing olanzapine improving long-term positive symptoms compared with typical antipsychotic drugs. Olanzapine showed a moderately positive effect on symptoms of depression compared with the typical antipsychotic drugs. Taking a conservative view, the authors report that the likelihood of premature study withdrawal was similar in each group. When odds ratios rather than relative risks were calculated, the likelihood of treatment dropout was shown to be lower in the olanzapine group at 3–12 months. Beyond 12 months the findings were equivocal (83% and 90% dropout in the olanzapine and typical antipsychotic-treated groups, respectively). There was no difference between olanzapine and the typical antipsychotic drugs over any time period when lack of efficacy was cited as a reason for leaving the study. In terms of tolerability, patients treated with olanzapine reported fewer anticholinergic side-effects (blurred vision, difficulty with urination). The olanzapine group required less concomitant anticholinergic medication than those taking haloperidol. There were significantly fewer EPS in the olanzapine-treated patients, across the range of symptoms (acute dystonia, parkinsonism, akathisia, hypokinesia and tremor). Weight gain was recorded as approximately 4kg over 3–12 months. The effects of olanzapine on quality of life, economic outcome, and cognitive function were all reported as 'not usable' by the authors. However, it was noted that a claim for improved cost-effectiveness of olanzapine over typical antipsychotic drugs was reported in one study. The authors report that data are missing on social functioning, employment status, death, and family satisfaction with care.

Two studies were cited, one of 8 weeks in duration with chlorpromazine as the comparator, and the other of 14 weeks' duration, comparing olanzapine with haloperidol. There was no difference between treatments in terms of clinical responses (though it is noted that the study comparing olanzapine with haloperidol reported significance in favour of olanzapine, but without reporting the actual data). There were no clinically significant differences between olanzapine and comparators in terms of positive or negative symptoms, total mental state or premature study withdrawal. Other adverse events reflected those reported for the large-scale studies above. Olanzapine was shown to be less likely to cause EPS in the study against chlorpromazine. No data were reported on quality of life, social functioning, employment, death and harm, cognitive functioning, satisfaction with treatment and cost-effectiveness.

Risperidone versus typical medication for schizophrenia

Kennedy et al (2000) compared risperidone with conventional antipsychotic drugs. All the available randomized controlled trials were included. Twelve short-term and two long-term studies were evaluated, providing data on 3401 patients. No evidence was, however, reported on the effect of risperidone on cognitive or social functioning, quality of life, employment status, discharge from hospital and relapse rates. Risperidone treatment increased the odds of moderate clinical improvement over conventional therapy. No additional effect on positive or negative symptoms of schizophrenia was noted. In comparison with haloperidol, there were significantly fewer movement disorders, and less need for concomitant anticholinergic medication. Risperidone treatment was associated with fewer dropouts and greater patient acceptability. Patients taking risperidone were less likely to experience somnolence but were more prone to weight gain. Analysis of the effect of risperidone dosing (excluding doses of 1–2mg) made little difference to the main outcome. Excluding data where the haloperidol dose was >10mg made no difference to risperidone's superiority with respect to EPS. The authors conclude that risperidone may be more acceptable to patients with schizophrenia, with 'marginal' benefits in terms of clinical improvement and side-effect profile compared with haloperidol. They suggested a possible publication bias in favour of risperidone, and proposed: 'Any marginal benefit should be balanced against the greater cost of the drug and its tendency to cause other effects such as weight gain'.

Quetiapine for schizophrenia

Srisurapanont et al (2000) evaluated all randomized controlled trials where quetiapine was compared with placebo, classic and other atypical antipsychotic drugs. Only those conclusions relating to comparisons of quetiapine against placebo and classic drugs will be discussed here. Eleven randomized controlled trials were included in the review. The number of participants per trial varied between 109 and 608, with the exception of two small studies sampling only 12 and 25 patients, respectively. The authors highlight the dropout rate of 36–64% in the 'short duration' trials and suggest that any outcome other than 'leaving the study early' should be viewed with caution, owing to the risk of bias incurred by the high dropout rate. In comparison to placebo, patients taking quetiapine were less likely to leave the study early, especially when the reason given was treatment failure. Quetiapine-treated patients also showed a significant improvement in psychotic symptoms compared to those receiving placebo. There was no difference from placebo in relation to the need for concomitant anticholinergic medication or for EPS effects.

In comparison to classic antipsychotic drugs, significantly fewer people in the quetiapine group left the study early. This effect was greater in the high-dose group and improvement in mental state was significantly better in the high-dose group. There were no differences between high- and low-dose groups in terms of akathisia, EPS or requirement for medication for extrapyramidal side-effects. There were no significant differences between the typical antipsychotic and quetiapine treatment groups with respect to mental state and global state. The authors called for larger, well conducted trials providing 'short, medium and long-term outcomes relevant to clinicians and carers'.

Amisulpride in the treatment of schizophrenia

The Cochrane Library did not contain any review of amisulpride. In the UK Royal College review of this drug, four short-term trials were identified including 603 patients. Three out of four trials demonstrated statistically significant improvements in symptom score compared with conventional antipsychotic drugs (though it is noted that doses of haloperidol in the trials were on the high side). There was an approximately 12% lower risk of dropping out of trials on amisulpride, and tolerability in terms of EPS was significantly greater in comparison with conventional therapy (National Schizophrenia Guideline Group, 1999). Leucht et al (2002) have performed a meta-analysis of 18 randomized controlled studies comparing amisulpride with conventional antipsychotic drugs ($n = 2214$). Amisulpride was more effective than conventional antipsychotic drugs, and its use was associated with significantly lower prescribing of antiparkinsonian medications and fewer dropouts.

Summary

✦ All clinical trials of atypical antipsychotic drugs may be criticized for their short duration and failure to provide indices that may be more relevant to overall longer-term outcome in schizophrenia.

✦ This criticism also applies to studies of sulpiride, loxapine and flupenthixol decanoate.

✦ Clozapine, olanzapine, risperidone, quetiapine and amisulpride were shown to be superior to placebo in terms of symptom reduction.

✦ All were less likely to cause movement disorders than typical antipsychotic drugs.

✦ Apart from clozapine (which did demonstrate therapeutic superiority to typical antipsychotic drugs), superiority to typical antipsychotic drugs in terms of symptom reduction was inconclusive both for positive and negative symptoms.

✦ Apart from clozapine, there is no proven difference in efficacy against positive and negative symptoms between different atypical antipsychotic drugs.

✦ Clozapine is the only atypical antipsychotic drug with proven efficacy in treatment-resistant schizophrenia.

✦ The cost-effectiveness of atypical antipsychotic drugs is established (see Taylor et al, 2002).

Weight gain and impaired glucose tolerance

Allison et al (1999) have attempted to retrospectively estimate and then compare the effects of antipsychotic drugs on body weight. They identified 81 English and non-English language articles providing data on weight change in patients treated with antipsychotic medication. Their research method included a computerized database search, and analysis of references obtained through the bibliographies of papers found; consultation, both with expert colleagues in the field and also authors of primary studies in order to ask for further references; requests to the manufacturer for both published and unpublished data relating to their respective compounds and weight gain; and perusal by interested parties to check for inaccuracies.

Meta-analysis and regression methods were used to provide an estimate of weight change after 10 weeks of treatment at a standard dose. The trials were also reviewed for qualitative information. The authors found that use of most antipsychotic drugs, conventional or atypical, was associated with weight gain. This was not attributable to placebo (patients on placebo lost weight). The greatest weight gain was associated with the use of clozapine and olanzapine, but it is notable that weight gain seen with these drugs was not significantly greater than that seen with the typical antipsychotic drugs chlorpromazine or thioridazine.

In discussing their findings, the authors touch on the clinical meaning of these degrees of weight gain. They point out that although their analysis is over only a 10-week period, where data were available for longer periods weight gain was even greater. Weight gain of >5% in the adult lifespan is associated with higher risks for endpoints such as mortality, cancer, cardiovascular disease, and diabetes. This implies that the weight gain associated with antipsychotic treatment (induced by both conventional and atypical antipsychotic drugs) may be clinically relevant. The authors go on to review potential strategies for managing weight gain, both pharmacological and non-pharmacological. These data have been substantiated in another systematic review (Taylor and McAskill, 2000), finding all atypical drugs with the exception of ziprasidone to be associated with weight gain.

Haupt and Newcomer (2001) review findings that type 2 diabetes mellitus and impaired glucose tolerance are associated with both typical and atypical antipsychotic treatment. These authors and more recent reviewers (Sernyak et al, 2002) agree the risk is increased for patients taking atypical antipsychotic medication. The strength of this association is greatest for chlorpromazine, clozapine and olanzapine. In the case of clozapine and olanzapine, the effect appears unrelated to adiposity. They suggest regular monitoring of weight, plasma glucose and lipid levels in patients taking antipsychotic medications.

QTc prolongation

Many antipsychotic drugs, perhaps a majority, have been shown to prolong the cardiac QT interval. In fact, methodological problems have meant that it is not yet possible to be sure that any antipsychotic does not affect the QT interval. QT prolongation may, in rare cases, give rise to the ventricular arrhythmia torsade de pointes, which is occasionally fatal. So far, only typical drugs have been clearly linked to torsade de pointes and increased cardiac mortality.

Although the risk to life is probably very small, some caution is advised when prescribing antipsychotics, both typical and atypical. In particular, the avoidance of antipsychotic polypharmacy is likely to reduce the risk of arrhythmia. ECG monitoring may be necessary in some cases (e.g. with typicals chlorpromazine and pimozide and with atypicals zotepine and sertindole) but only where there are other risk factors present (e.g. cardiac disease, electrolyte disturbance, use of inhibitors of antipsychotic metabolism). The QT interval is notoriously difficult to measure and interpret. Therefore, ECG monitoring is perhaps best performed by a specialist cardiologist. Overall, the aim should be to avoid the need for ECG monitoring by using single antipsychotics in low doses while avoiding metabolic interaction (Taylor, 2002).

Conventional vs novel antipsychotic drugs – a recent naturalistic study of subjective tolerability, side-effects and impact on quality of life

The Cochrane reviewers frequently call for longer-term, naturalistic data that provide indices meaningful to both individual patients and the wider community. The subjective acceptance of a drug by patients is key to ensuring compliance, the major factor in relapse prevention. Voruganti and colleagues (2000) partially address this issue. A total of 230 patients, divided into five comparable groups stabilized on conventional antipsychotic drugs, risperidone, olanzapine, quetiapine or clozapine for a period of 6 months or longer, were cross-sectionally evaluated. A community-based schizophrenia research programme affiliated with a university teaching hospital provided the setting for the study. The choice of drug and the dose prescribed was independent of the research team. 'Clinical stability' was defined as a lack of exacerbation of symptoms or need for hospitalization in the 6-month period prior to the evaluation. The results showed that patients receiving novel antipsychotic drugs experienced fewer side-effects and reported more positive subjective responses and favourable attitudes toward their treatment. The patients on novel antipsychotic drugs also had a lower prevalence of what these authors designated 'neuroleptic dysphoria', reflecting persistent subjective unhappiness due to the drug. To date, this side-effect of antipsychotic medication has not been widely discussed. It is being increasingly recognized in the literature, and could be an important cause of non-adherence (as well as an iatrogenic contribution to depression in schizophrenic patients). Importantly, this effect does not run in parallel with clinical response, and the authors defined some individuals as 'dysphoric responders'. The proportion of these patients was significantly greater in the group treated with conventional antipsychotic drugs. Self-rated quality of life was also significantly better in patients on atypical antipsychotic drugs. These data – explicitly assessing subjective tolerability, side-effects and quality of life – support the implicit suggestion from clinical trials data, that fewer side-effects should lead to better tolerated drugs and greater patient satisfaction. Of further relevance is the finding, by the same group (Norman et al, 2000), that positive and negative symptoms and functional levels correlate with quality of life ratings, but that positive symptoms are particularly associated with general well-being.

Naber (1995) has also studied subjective well-being in patients on the atypical drug clozapine. Forty patients on clozapine were compared with 40 patients on haloperidol or flupenthixol. There was a significant improvement in subjective well-being in patients treated with clozapine. This paper also highlights the importance of emotional and cognitive effects of typical antipsychotic therapy on the quality of life of a chronically treated patient's quality of life. A high level of patient satisfaction with clozapine, as opposed to classic antipsychotic medication, has also been reported by Taylor et al (2000).

Stanniland and Taylor (2000) have reviewed the relative tolerability of atypical antipsychotic drugs. They conclude that as well as weight gain, anticholinergic, sedative and hypotensive effects do occur (to a variable extent) with these drugs, and this is associated with withdrawals from short-term clinical trials. Nevertheless, they also make the distinct and important observation of a decline in serious adverse events, with atypical drugs showing clear superiority over typical agents. These include hyperprolactinaemia, tardive dyskinesia and EPS. In their view, 'to prescribe typical drugs is perhaps, based on comparative data…to do harm when a suitable alternative is available'.

Is low-dose conventional antipsychotic treatment an alternative to atypical antipsychotic treatment?

Taylor (2000) has discussed the concept of using low-dose typical medication instead of an atypical antipsychotic, as suggested by the UK Royal College Guidelines. Taking the recommended 12mg or less of haloperidol, it is possible to evaluate whether these doses could induce EPS or hyperprolactinaemia. In this context, it is worth bearing in mind the PET data in the study by Kapur et al (1999). This confirms that doses as low as 2mg of haloperidol produce high striatal D2 occupancy levels predictive of both elevated prolactin levels and EPS. Furthermore, in an Italian survey of 1559 patients, in whom >75% were taking ≤10mg of haloperidol equivalents, approximately one third experienced EPS and a fifth had persistent tardive dyskinesia (Muscoletta et al, 1999). More recent studies also show that the therapeutic and EPS effects of fluphenazine and haloperidol cannot be separated by dose (Levinson et al, 1990; Rifkin et al, 1991). Another study attempted to define the threshold dose for the appearance of EPS effects in first-episode and relapsed schizophrenic patients (McEvoy et al, 1991). Patients were given haloperidol 2mg and the dose was increased either until rigidity appeared or worsened, or until a dose of 10mg was reached (there was dose reduction to 1mg or 0.5mg if rigidity appeared at the 2mg dose). Those previously exposed to neuroleptics required 4.3 (0.5–10)mg/day before the appearance of EPS, while for first-episode patients the dose was lower, i.e. 2.1 (0.5–4)mg/day. These doses were associated with clinical benefit, but the important point is that there was no window between the desired and the unwanted effects of the drug. Furthermore, a large (n = 500) prospective, randomized double-blind comparison of different doses of haloperidol compared to sertindole (an atypical antipsychotic drug) and placebo showed that even subtherapeutic doses of haloperidol could produce EPS effects (Zimbroff et al, 1997). One small, open-label (no comparator used) study of haloperidol (dose <1mg) in first-episode patients showed good response with few EPS emergent, but clearly dosing was within a narrow therapeutic window (Oosthuizen et al, 2001)

Summary

✦ Like typical antipsychotic drugs, atypical compounds induce a variety of side-effects.

✦ Patients receiving any antipsychotic drug should be regularly monitored with respect to weight and plasma glucose (6-monthly at least, and more often with clozapine or olanzapine).

✦ By definition, atypical drugs are qualitatively different from classic drugs, with an intrinsic tendency to low EPS (and tardive dyskinesia).

✦ Service users may now be offered more choice and appear more satisfied with atypical antipsychotic medication.

4 Running a medication review service

In order to make clinically sound judgements about future treatment, it is essential to obtain an accurate and comprehensive account of the patient's present and past circumstances. Particular attention needs to be paid to details of treatment (past and present), including response and side-effects. A holistic approach to information gathering was adopted, using as many sources as possible to cross-reference, collate and corroborate accounts obtained from the patient. To achieve this, we used a systematic approach, and implemented the principles of evidence-based practice by ensuring that every patient was clinically rated for symptoms and side-effects, and that corresponding physical measures were recorded.

All patients were assessed by means of a:

✦   Full psychiatric history

✦   Thorough case note review

✦   Brief interview with carers and/or keyworker

✦   Full battery of rating scales, aimed at providing a quantitative assessment of psychiatric symptoms and side-effects

✦   Routine nursing physical examination (temperature, pulse, blood pressure, ECG, weight, height and body mass index (BMI))

✦   Full laboratory blood tests:

     – Urea and electrolytes

     – Liver function tests

     – Thyroid function tests

     – Blood glucose and cholesterol

     – Full blood count

     – Serum prolactin

     – Current drug plasma levels – not generally available in reliable form for the majority of drugs (see section later)

✦   Urinalysis and urine culture and sensitivity (C and S).

Full psychiatric history

This is the established format for comprehensive and systematic psychiatric assessment. The full psychiatric history provides a framework for interviewing and enables fluid and intuitive progression of the interview. It includes all the tools necessary to make an assessment of current clinical condition, risk, and diagnosis. For full psychiatric history, see Appendix III.

Case note review

Although this is time-consuming, it nearly always yields valuable information that otherwise would not have been obtained. In many instances, the medication history provided by the patient – often spanning many years' duration – is incomplete or inaccurate, and memories of responses to various treatments are unreliable. Specific entries in the case notes sometimes highlight aspects of patients' symptoms that may prompt a re-evaluation of the diagnosis, and so be used to inform decisions about future care and treatment.

Brief interview with carer or keyworker

This is another invaluable tool for assessing current clinical condition and response to current and past treatments. These interviews are useful for both corroborating and raising questions about the patient's account of past and present circumstances.

Rating scales

Rating scales are a quantitative measure of current clinical condition and response to treatment. The 'scoring' system of the scale provides a reference point for future consultations and assessments. This type of assessment fulfils the remit of evidence-based practice and is a systematic and thorough method of recording baseline measurements and evaluating outcome. A full battery of rating scales covering a wide spectrum of symptoms, side-effects, social functioning and service use/provision was employed. The list of scales appears below; actual scales can be found in Appendix II

Performing the rating scales is an acquired skill. It is recommended that all staff intending to use them are trained in their administration. Inter-rater reliability is an essential requirement if teams are to integrate regular ratings into their clinical practice.

The recommended method of ensuring inter-rater reliability is that teams either practise rating live patients, or that they acquire videotapes of interviews, which they observe together as a team. Each team member makes an individual assessment, and at the end of the session, the team discuss the case and compare scores. A flipchart is a useful tool, as individual scores can be displayed, discussed and compared. Where there is dissent about an individual item on a scale, each team member's rationale for his/her scoring method can be discussed. Generally speaking, a discrepancy of 1 point on a scale of 1–7 is not significant; however, if consistently significant discrepancies occur amongst team members, it is important that extra time be taken to ensure that:

✦ The rating process is fully understood

✦ The wording of the score rationale (provided with scale) is fully understood

✦ Each team member has sufficient expertise to administer the scale.

List of scales used

(The scales appear in Appendix II, which begins on p.61.)

+ PANSS (Positive and Negative Symptom Scale) (Kay et al, 1987)

+ BPRS (Brief Psychiatric Rating Scale) (Overall and Gorham, 1962)

+ CGI (Clinical Global Impression) (Guy, 1976)

+ GAS (Global Assessment Scale) (Endicott et al, 1976)

+ HONOS (Health of the Nation Outcome Scale) (Wing et al, 1998)

+ Calgary Depression Scale (Addington et al, 1993)

+ Schizophrenia Quality of Life Scale (Wilkinson et al, 2000)

+ Simpson–Angus Scale (Simpson and Angus, 1970)

+ Barnes Akathisia Scale (Barnes, 1989)

+ AIMS (Abnormal Involuntary Movements Scale) (Wiener and Lang, 1995)

+ LUNSERS (Liverpool University Side-effects Rating Scale) (Day et al, 1995)

+ SFQ (Sexual Functioning Questionnaire) (Smith et al, 2002)

+ Sexual Dysfunction Checklist (Lingjaerde, 2002)

+ Client Service Receipt Inventory (Beecham and Knapp, 1992)

+ DAI-10 (Drug Attitude Inventory) (Hogan et al, 1983)

+ UKU Side-effects Scale (Lingjaerde, 1987)

Routine nursing physical examination

The routine nursing physical (comprising temperature, blood pressure, pulse, electrocardiograph (ECG), weight, and BMI (which requires a height measurement) should be routinely undertaken on all psychiatric patients at least 6-monthly.

BMI: (Body Mass Index)

This is a standardized measure of healthy weight based on height:weight ratio. The BMI is obtained using the following formula: weight (kg)/height (m^2). The BMI was originally intended to be used as an indicator of potential weight-related morbidity and risk probability and has long been used by life insurance companies as such. As BMI is a pure measure of weight, and does not take body composition into account, it can be unreliable as an indicator of healthy weight in some circumstances, particularly when arbitrarily applied. Ethnic and gender-related variations in body composition may skew weight:height ratios. African/Caribbean people generally have a heavier musculature and bone mass than Caucasian and Asian people, and thus tend to weigh more, though they may have a lower body fat percentage than Caucasian/Asian people. They may therefore have a higher BMI without associated health risks. Men have a higher muscle:fat ratio than women, so will also have a higher BMI without associated health risks. A more accurate measure of measuring health/morbidity risk is the waist:hip ratio (WHR) which measures the waist circumference (cm):hip circumference (cm). The WHR is a measure of abdominal obesity, a clear risk factor for several physical conditions, including cardiovascular disease and non-insulin-dependent diabetes mellitus (NIDDM).

The standard measurements for BMI as a corollary of health are:

✦ 19–25: healthy weight

✦ 25–30: overweight

✦ 30–35: obese

✦ >35: morbidly obese (various categories exist for BMI >35).

ECG

Many antipsychotic drugs alter the QTc interval, with potentially fatal consequences. Patients commencing antipsychotic treatment, switching to some antipsychotic medications, or taking more than one antipsychotic drug should have a baseline ECG (see earlier section relating to QTc interval).

Risks for altered QTc intervals are in roughly the following order:

Moderate risk: Pimozide, zotepine, thioridazine

Mild–moderate risk: Quetiapine, haloperidol, risperidone, clozapine, chlorpromazine, depot preparations.

Laboratory blood tests

These tests should be taken on all psychiatric patients at least yearly, and in many cases more frequently than this. It is recommended that :

✦ Patients taking atypical antipsychotics have blood glucose and triglycerides measured 6-monthly or at any time if symptoms suggest a high index of suspicion (Henderson et al, 2000; Mir and Taylor, 2001; Sernyak et al, 2002).

✦ Patients taking lithium should have 6-monthly urea and electrolytes (U & E) and thyroid function tests and lithium levels.

For a list of normal blood values, see Appendix I.

5 Medication review services in the community

The Care Programme Approach (CPA) is the accepted framework for caring for people with severe mental illness in the community. The CPA is a holistic model and encompasses all the aspects of clinical and social management necessary to ensure that the patient remains as mentally and functionally well as possible. The formal framework of the CPA addresses:

✦   Current and past clinical condition

✦   Proposed input from mental health services

✦   Relapse indicators

✦   The patient's relationships and support structures

✦   Social and financial circumstances

✦   Medication.

In mainstream mental health services, medication remains the mainstay of treatment. Under the CPA, facilitating adherence to medication regimens is a requirement of mental health clinicians. Community mental health teams (CMHTs) should offer medication services that facilitate adherence to medication. This means using thorough, regular and systematic review of all patients as regards:

✦   Treatment regimens

✦   Clinical condition

✦   Side-effects

✦   Physical health

with a view to optimizing clinical and functional condition and minimizing side-effects and other potential confounds to adherence.

The use of standardized rating scales and systematic physical examinations is an essential tool in assessing baseline status and charting progress, particularly if patients may be receiving medication and treatment from a variety of sources. Community patients may variously receive treatment from:

✦   GP surgery

✦   Community mental health team base

✦   Depot clinic

✦   Outpatient clinic

+ General or psychiatric hospital A&E clinic

+ In their own home, from a keyworker.

Where treatment is disseminated, standardized assessments are the only accurate method of quantitatively evaluating clinical condition, progress, efficacy and tolerability of treatment. Many community patients are stably maintained on treatment, but suffer side-effects or residual psychotic symptoms that are not identified because of:

+ Time constraints

+ Low staffing levels

+ The patient's appearance of stability

+ Lack of any systematized regular review service.

Most CMHTs already have a medication service in the form of a depot clinic. The majority of patients engaged with depot clinics attend regularly, are reasonably clinically stable, and rarely cause concern. This means, however, that there often appears to be little cause for review, and as a result, many of them may be taking medication that only partially suppresses their symptoms and/or causes unacceptable side-effects, i.e. the patient may be stable but still sick.

Aims of a community medication service

+ To provide an opportunity for every patient to have a thorough psychiatric and physical review.

+ To offer every patient the opportunity to conduct a dialogue about their treatment options.

+ To offer every patient the opportunity to receive information about the best possible treatment.

+ To identify side-effects and residual symptomatology and treat appropriately.

+ To do all the above in a systematic, evidence-based manner.

Setting up a community medication service

In most areas, established depot clinics will already exist. Setting up a medication review clinic involves modifying the existing resource to provide a more acceptable service to patients.

Basic requirements before setting up

1. Formulation of local clinic policy and protocols after discussion with all community personnel.
2. Formulation of policy about modes of referral between medication review service, CMHT and local primary care providers.
3. Distribution of written procedural guidelines to all medication review clinic and local CMHT staff, including the advertising of clinic times and referral mode.
4. Ensuring clarity regarding lines of responsibility for prescribing, administering medication and ongoing follow-up of the patients.
5. Establishing lines of communication according to local protocol. It is usual to ensure that no decisions/changes are made without the responsible team's involvement and agreement. This is best achieved by documenting all relevant information in the patient's notes.

Setting up

✦ Deciding on a comprehensive ratings package, and ensuring inter-rater reliability within the service.

✦ Identifying and equipping suitable space for the clinic (a consulting room and a clinical examination room).

✦ Requirements for clinical examination room:

– Medicine cabinet

– Designated physical examination area with couch

– Accurate weighing scales and height measure

– ECG machine

– Sphygmomanometer (with standard and outsize cuffs)

– Thermometers

– Standard neurological tray

– Phlebotomy equipment (tourniquets, variety of needles and syringes, cotton wool, plasters, swabs, supply of all standard blood collection bottles and request forms)

– Equipment for collecting and testing urine.

Staffing

+ Clinic nurses – the number of nurses needed for the clinic will depend on the population served and the numbers of patients on long-term antipsychotic medication. For a population of approximately 1000 patients with severe mental illness, two nurses should be sufficient to run the clinic. This number assumes that some patients will continue to receive their medication from other sources, but will attend the medication clinic for review on a 1–2-yearly basis. The clinic nurses should ideally be trained at 'F' grade or above, and able to administer all the relevant rating scales and examinations, as well as being experienced in clinical assessment.

+ Doctor – this should be a senior SHO or specialist registrar, who will be able to conduct physical examinations and carry out the medication review in addition to the nurses.

+ Senior psychiatrist in a consultative role.

Logistics

+ Clarifying and agreeing on the time commitment available from clinic staff: the Maudsley Medication Review Service provided three sessions/week over 1 day, using three staff members.

+ Advertising the service: a leaflet providing information about the service objectives, location, referral mode and interventions was devised, printed and distributed. Separate leaflets were printed for clinicians and service users.

The clinic then began accepting referrals from doctors and community mental health workers.

The clinic in practice

+ Assessments took 2–3 hours face-to face and a further 3–4 hours for writing up.

+ After assessing patients, the cases were presented at the medication review team meeting (weekly), and an opinion as to the best treatment option was generated.

+ All correspondence was sent to the sector team and the GP.

The medication review clinic team then awaited the response from the sector consultant psychiatrist as to whether we should proceed with the specified treatment option.

6 The pro-forma

MEDICATION REVIEW CLINIC
• **List of personnel**
Address for correspondence:

Dr
Consultant Psychiatrist

Date:

Dear Dr,

Re:

Mr/Ms   attended the medication review clinic on   . A full assessment including physical examination, laboratory bloods, urinalysis and rating scales was performed.

Diagnosis:
1.

Current treatment:

I reviewed Mr/Ms   personally and examined the medical notes to establish the following information:

Current complaints:

History of presenting complaints

Past psychiatric history:

Drug history:
Compliance history:

Risk and forensic history:
Self-harm:
Harm to others:

Personal history:

Family history:

Past medical history:

Allergies:

Social circumstances:

Habits:

Mental health services:

Today on **mental state examination:**

A & B:
Speech:
Mood:
Thoughts:
Perceptions:
Cognition:
Insight:

Physical examination:
Cardiovascular, respiratory, abdominal and neurological examinations:
Weight: kg
Height: m   BMI:
BP: /
HR: reg.

Blood test results

Prolactin (mU/l)	
TSH (mU/l)	
Na (mmol/l)	
K (mmol/l)	
Ur (mmol/l)	
Cr (mmol/l)	
Glucose (mmol/l)	
Bilirubin (mmol/l)	
Alk phos (IU/l)	
ALT (IU/l)	
AST (IU/l)	
GGT (IU/l)	
ALB (g/l)	
Calcium (corrected) (mmol/l)	
Cholesterol (mmol/l)	
Hb	
Urine: C & S	

Formulation:
Mr/Ms   is a   year-old man/woman who lives in a   . He/she has a   year history of   . He/she has been admitted to hospital for   times, on   occasions under the MHA. His/her positive symptoms have   to antipsychotic medication.

Risk assessment:
To self:
To others:
Of relapse:

Opinion:
After reviewing Mr/Ms   and discussing all of the above at our team meeting, we have formed the following opinion:

We are happy to offer monitoring and pro-active follow-up for the switch. We leave it to the community team's discretion as to whether they consider this the best course of action.

We look forward to receiving the team's decision.

Yours sincerely,

See Appendix I for rating scale results
Cc: CPN, GP

Appendix I

Rating scales
General functioning

	Rating	Comments
GAS	(1 (min) – 100 (max.))	Level of functioning and impairment:
CGI	(1 (least ill) – 7 (most ill))	Overall compared to patients with similar illness:
HONOS	(1 (least problems – 108 (most problems)	Impact of mental illness:
Schizophrenia Quality of Life Scale	Rating : 0 (good quality of life) – 100 (poor quality of life) Psychological: Energy/motivation: Symptoms/side-effects	

Mental state

	Rating	Comments
PANNS – positive	0–60	
PANNS – negative	0–60	
PANNS – composite		
PANNS – general	0–60	
PANNS – overall	0–180	
BPRS*	0–114	
MMSE	/30	
Calgary Depression	/27	

* Two versions of the BPRS scale exist: a 24-item scale that measures individual symptoms on a scale of 1–7, and a newer 18-item scale that measures individual symptoms on a scale of 0–6. The Medication Review Service uses the 18-item scale

Medication side-effects and compliance

	Rating	Comments
UKU – psychic	(0 (min) –30 (max))	
UKU – neuro	(0 (min) –24 (max))	
UKU – autonomic	(0 (min) –33 (max))	
UKU – other	(0 (min) –57 (max))	
Angus–Simpson	0–36	
AIMS	0–42	
Barnes Akathisia	0–14	
Sex Function Qst	Concerns or otherwise	
Compliance Qst	(range: −12 − +12)	
Drug Attitude Inventory	(−10–+10)	

7 Sample case study

Re: John DOE, d.o.b 01/01/69

Mr Doe attended the medication review clinic on 1 December. A full assessment, including physical examination, laboratory bloods, urinalysis and rating scales, was performed.

Diagnosis:
1. Paranoid schizophrenia

Current treatment:
Flupenthixol decanoate 200mg 2-weekly
Procyclidine 10mg BD
Haloperidol 5mg prn

Mr Doe was reviewed personally and the medical notes examined to establish the following information:

Current complaints:

✦   Stiff muscles (from patient: ' I feel stiff and sore all the time')

✦   Sexual dysfunction (loss of libido, erectile dysfunction) (from patient: ' I hardly ever feel like sex any more, and even when I do, it's hard to get an erection')

History of presenting complaints:

Mr Doe has suffered from dystonia for several years (since starting treatment with antipsychotic medication in 1994). His erectile dysfunction and loss of libido have become more apparent since he and his partner decided they would like to have a child last year.

Past psychiatric history:
From patient: First became ill in 1994, aged 25. Describes the onset of his illness as quite sudden – became convinced that he was being followed, and his work telephone bugged. Accused colleagues of harassment, and became abusive and violent at work. Was admitted to the Maudsley Hospital.

From case notes:
January 1994: Patient was brought into hospital on a Section 136 after causing a disturbance at work (smashing a colleague's computer screen and attempting to strangle him). Had apparently been behaving oddly for about a week prior to this, staring into space and at colleagues, not eating or sleeping, and arriving at and leaving work at odd times of the day. Two days prior to admission, had been found going through a colleague's filing cabinet at 1am. Possible precipitating factors were:

✦   Heavy use of cannabis and alcohol for about 2 weeks prior to admission

✦   Had broken up with his girlfriend of 2 years just before Christmas

✦   Had missed out on a promotion at work he had been expecting.

While in hospital, presented with persecutory delusions (being followed, photographed and 'got at' by people at work and MI5), and hallucinations (a voice calling his name, and 'buzzing' noises). Treated with haloperidol, improved and was discharged after 3 weeks.

September 1994: Presented at the Emergency Clinic complaining that he thought he might be under surveillance again. Had recently stopped medication as he felt it was impairing his concentration. Managed as an outpatient, recommenced on medication, and soon stabilized.

January 1996: Presented for outpatient appointment as fearful and upset. Felt he was becoming ill again. Meds increased.

March 1998: Admitted to Maudsley hospital on Section 136 after breaking into (absent) neighbour's house and dismantling light fittings. Neighbour had arrived home and called police. Patient apparently 'looking for bugs and cameras'. While in hospital became depressed and suicidal, as feared he would lose job. Meds changed, antidepressant added, soon stabilized. This admission 8 weeks.

May 1998 – present: Stable.

Drug history:

January 1994: Treated in hospital with haloperidol 10mg/day, responded rapidly. Developed mild dystonia, procyclidine 5mg BD added with some effect.

September 1994: Medication changed to haloperidol decanoate 100mg 2 weekly IM as patient had stopped oral meds. Dystonia worsened, procyclidine increased to 10mg BD.

January 1996: Haloperidol decanoate increased to 150mg 2-weekly IM as patient becoming ill (fearful, agitated) Responded well, no increase in side-effects noted.

March 1998: Meds changed to flupenthixol decanoate 200mg 2 weekly IM after relapse. Patient complained of dystonia, procyclidine continued. Given some haloperidol 5mg tablets as PRN medication in case of impending relapse.

Patient feeling actively suicidal during admission – commenced on fluoxetine 20mg mane with good effect.

December 1998: Stable with no psychotic symptoms. Stated at outpatient appointment that he had stopped fluoxetine in September, with no worsening of mood. Wife (in attendance) felt he was managing well without it. Patient and wife agreed to contact CMHT and recommence fluoxetine if signs of depression reappeared. Has been relatively stable on this regimen since.

Compliance history:

Initially poor compliance with oral medication, and compliance improved when switched to depot. Now is saying he cannot bear the side-effects of his medication (flupenthixol) and would like to switch. Says he will take oral meds as he is aware he needs medication to prevent relapse.

Risk and forensic history:

Self harm: Mild risk – has felt suicidal in the past, but never made an attempt. Denies active or passive suicidal ideation at present.

Harm to others: No history of violence prior to becoming mentally ill. Has assaulted colleagues and police in the past as a direct result of his illness. While stable on medication, presents little risk.

Forensic history: Nil.

Personal history:

Born in London. Normal birth, normal milestones. Was a happy child, enjoyed school, did well in exams. Left school at 18 with 3 'A' Levels, did Media Studies at X Polytechnic, majored in Creative Writing. Worked for a publishing firm for 2 years, then left and joined a smaller company with 'better opportunities'. Had first breakdown after a year in this job. Had a year off work, then in 1995 went to work in X branch of Waterstones (part time) – has worked there since.

Met wife (Jane) on a Waterstones training course in 1999, married in 2000. She has a daughter (aged 8) from a previous relationship. Couple have been trying to conceive for the last year.

Relationship generally good, but has become strained of late due to patient's sexual problems.

Family history:
Mother died last year (ca breast) Father a judge, alive and well; is about to remarry. Patient middle child of three. Two sisters, both well, married with children, 'have done well in their careers'. Patient has a good relationship with father and sisters ('They have all been very good to me').
Maternal grandmother had 'some sort of mental illness' (committed suicide), one maternal aunt (also dead) 'in and out of mental hospitals all her life'. No other F/H of mental illness.

Past medical history:
Nil significant
Allergies: Nil known

Social circumstances:
Lives with wife and stepdaughter in own house in X. Pleasant accommodation. Wife works part-time in a local bookshop. Patient works part-time in a West End branch of Waterstones. Patient and wife share child care. No current money problems. Patient tends to spend most of spare time with family, or working on the house and garden. Has a few friends, but doesn't go out much.

Habits:
Cigarette smoker – about 20/day
Alcohol: a few beers at the weekend
Illicit drugs: nil now – used to smoke cannabis, hasn't done so for about 5 years. Had tried cocaine once or twice before he became ill.

Mental health services:
Sees a psychiatrist in outpatients once every 6 months. Attends depot clinic for medication every 2 weeks. Has no CPN, does not attend a day centre.

Today on **mental state examination:**
A & B: Pleasant, well-groomed Caucasian man of stated age. Good rapport and eye contact, clear historian.
Speech: Normal rate, flow and volume. No formal thought disorder.
Mood: Appears euthymic, able to smile, and laughed on one (appropriate) occasion. Denies passive or active suicidal ideation, but acknowledges that he occasionally feels 'quite low'. Adamant that he does not want antidepressants.
Thoughts: Occasionally, when feeling stressed, wonders whether it's 'all starting up again', but is able to convince self that 'it's not real'. Takes some PRN haloperidol whenever this happens.
Perceptions: Appear normal, denies hallucinations.
Cognition: Not formally tested but appears grossly intact. Scored 30/30 in MMSE (Mini Mental State Examination, Folstein et al, 1975).
Insight: Good. Acknowledges that he has a mental illness, and needs regular medication.

Physical examination:
Cardiovascular, respiratory, abdominal and neurological examinations: no abnormalities noted.
Weight: 84kg
Height: 1.82m   BMI: 25.3
BP: 130/85
HR: 72 reg.

Blood test results:

(For normal ranges, see Appendix I)

Prolactin (mU/l)	782 * high
TSH (mU/l)	2.6
Na (mmol/l)	138
K (mmol/l)	4.7
Ur (mmol/l)	4.4
Cr (mmol/l)	98
Glucose (mmol/l)	5.1
Bilirubin (mmol/l)	11
Alk phos (IU/l)	78
ALT (IU/l)	29
AST (IU/l)	18
GGT (IU/l)	22
ALB (g/l)	43
Calcium (corrected) (mmol/l)	2.4
Cholesterol (mmol/l)	4.8
Hb	15.2
Urine: ketones or glucose	NAD

Formulation:
Mr Doe is a 32-year-old man who lives with his wife and stepdaughter in their own house. He has a 7-year history of paranoid schizophrenia with occasional bouts of depression. He has been admitted to hospital twice, on both occasions under the MHA. His positive symptoms have responded well to flupenthixol, but he has been left with some residual negative symptoms. He has always experienced extrapyramidal side-effects from his antipsychotic medication, such that he has always needed to take regular anticholinergic drugs. More recently, he has developed problems with his sexual functioning which are causing marital tension. He and his wife would like to conceive a child, but he is currently unable to have full intercourse. He would like to change his medication.

His current mental state is stable, and although he admits to feeling 'low' at times, he is not clinically depressed and presents no risk to himself or others at present.

Risk assessment:
To self: nil or very minor risk while mentally well and taking medication
To others: nil or very minor risk while mentally well and taking medication
Of relapse: very strong risk if he stops medication, mild–moderate risk otherwise.

Opinion:
Mr Doe has responded well to flupenthixol, but tolerates it poorly. In view of his sexual problems and his persistent extrapyramidal side-effects – both of which are very distressing to him – we would recommend that he switch to a prolactin-sparing agent such as olanzapine or quetiapine, which is very unlikely to cause the same problems even across the full dosing range. We note that his serum prolactin is raised, but would expect this to normalize and his sexual problems to at least partially resolve within 8–10 weeks of stopping depot medication. We suggest that he commence quetiapine a week before his depot is due in order to achieve cross-titration and maintain adequate antipsychotic cover, and that his procyclidine is slowly withdrawn over a period of a month.

Mr Doe's mental state should be monitored closely during the switching period, and his wife alerted to the need to watch out for signs of relapse.

We are happy to offer monitoring and proactive follow-up for the switch. We leave it to the community team's discretion as to whether they consider this the best course of action.

We look forward to receiving the team's decision.
Yours sincerely,

See Appendix I for rating scale results
cc, CPN, GP

Appendix I

Rating scales

General functioning

	Rating	Comments
GAS	70 (1 (min) –100 (max))	Level of functioning and impairment: some mild symptoms, but generally functioning pretty well, has some meaningful interpersonal relationships and most untrained people would not consider him 'sick'
CGI	2 (1 (least ill) –7 (most ill))	Overall compared to patients with similar illness: borderline
HONOS	3 (1 (least problems–108 (most problems)	Impact of mental illness: minor, non-clinical problem with depressed mood, anxiety and relationships
SQLS	0–100 for 3 subscales: • Psychological • Energy/motivation • Symptoms/side-effects • For all subscales, 0 denotes good quality of life and 100 denotes poor quality of life	Psychological: 42 – significantly impaired Energy/motivation: 25 – moderately impaired Symptoms/side-effects: 31.3 – moderately to significantly impaired

Mental State

	Rating	Comments
PANNS – positive	8	Virtually asymptomatic, very slightly suspicious
PANNS – negative	10	Very slight affective blunting and social withdrawal
PANNS – composite	−2	Slightly negative presentation
PANNS – general	20	Scored 3 for depression and anxiety
PANNS- overall	38	Stable at present
BPRS	32	Scored 3 for depression and anxiety
MMSE	30/30	No gross cognitive impairment detected
Calgary Depression	3/27	Mildly depressed

Medication side-effects and compliance

	Rating	Comments
UKU – psychic	6 (min)–30 (max))	Tension and inner unrest, depression and concentration difficulties; almost certainly due to medication
UKU – neuro	7 (min)–24 (max))	Dystonia and mild tremor, rigidity; almost certainly due to medication
UKU – autonomic	1 (min)–33 (max))	Mild dryness of mouth; almost certainly due to medication
UKU – other	6 (min) –57 (max))	Sexual dysfunction; almost certainly due to medication
Angus–Simpson	8	Moderate limb stiffness, mild tremor
AIMS	0	No abnormal movements
Barnes Akathisia	3	No observed akathisia, but subjectively present
Sex Function Qst	Concerns	Moderate loss of libido and erectile dysfunction causing problems within current relationship
Compliance Qst	Range: −12 –+12	4 – good compliance – feels he needs medication, but that this is the wrong medication for him
Drug Attitude Inventory	(−10–+10)	8 – good compliance – acknowledges side-effects

8 A guide to drug interactions and successful switching

Drug interactions fall broadly into two categories:

+ Pharmacodynamic: the effects of these interactions are generally additive, brought about by one drug being added to another, or increased potentiation of drug effects at the neuroreceptor level.

+ Pharmacokinetic: these effects include metabolic inhibition or induction at a cellular level (Taylor, 1997).

Most common interaction situations

Polypharmacy (prescribed or otherwise)
Cross-titration during a switch

+ Atypical antipsychotics with conventional antipsychotics

+ Atypical antipsychotics with other atypicals

+ Atypical antipsychotics and other psychotropic agents, e.g. mood stabilizers

+ Acute situations: conventional antipsychotic/atypical antipsychotic/sedative drugs

+ Clozapine and other antipsychotic drugs

Monotherapy is ideal, but sometimes untenable – particularly when:
a) cross-titrating
b) in acute situations
c) there is an affective component to psychosis

---

9 Interactions

Atypical and conventional antipsychotic agents

✦ Look for potentiation of side-effects – orthostatic hypotension, anticholinergic effects, sedation – when mixing low-potency antipsychotics like chlorpromazine and clozapine or quetiapine.

✦ Thioridazine (withdrawn for new prescription in UK, but still in occasional use) may reduce quetiapine levels, but increase other drug levels.

✦ Some antipsychotics (especially phenothiazines and flupenthixol) may increase risk of neutropenia when added to clozapine.

✦ Potential for lowering of seizure threshold when using clozapine, loxapine, zotepine or chlorpromazine alone or together.

✦ Appearance or worsening of extrapyramidal side-effects when using conventional neuroleptics with risperidone, amisulpride, or when using high-dose olanzapine ($\geqslant$20mg), amisulpride (> 800mg) or risperidone (> 6mg).

Atypical vs atypical drug interactions

✦ Most common when cross-titrating during a switch.

✦ Reports of sudden rise in clozapine levels and agranulocytosis when risperidone was added to clozapine.

✦ Reports of weight loss when olanzapine/quetiapine were combined with clozapine.

✦ Potential for increased risk of sedation and orthostatic hypotension when using clozapine, quetiapine or olanzapine in any combination.

Atypicals and other psychotropic agents

Olanzapine

✦ Some interaction with benzodiazepines – mild increase in heart rate, dry mouth and sedation reported.

✦ Carbamazepine reduces half-life of olanzapine by 20% and increases clearance by 44%.

✦ Lithium or sodium valproate: may contribute to weight gain.

Risperidone

- Carbamazepine: an increase in risperidone clearance in chronic use.

- Clozapine: two cases of raised clozapine levels (one by 73%; the other patient developed agranulocytosis).

- Lithium: single case report of delirium; single case report of NMS.

- Lithium or sodium valproate: may contribute to weight gain.

Quetiapine

- Lithium: quetiapine may increase lithium levels slightly – quetiapine may also rarely affect thyroid function.

- Carbamazepine: may lower quetiapine levels slightly.

- Barbiturates: may lower quetiapine levels slightly.

- Lithium or sodium valproate: may contribute to weight gain.

Clozapine

- Other antipsychotics: may increase risk of neutropenia.

- Anticholinergics: increased antimuscarinic effects.

- Benzodiazepines: increased sedation and may cause respiratory depression.

- MAOIs, alcohol, opioids: respiratory depression.

- SSRIs may increase clozapine levels (especially fluvoxamine – citalopram and nefazodone have negligible if any effect).

- Antibiotics: some may increase risk of neutropenia.

- Antihypertensives: will lower BP further.

- Warfarin and digoxin: clozapine increases effects.

- Phenytoin: lowers clozapine levels.

- Cimetidine: raises clozapine levels.

- Mood stabilizers:

  - carbamazepine may increase risk of neutropenia

  - lithium may increase risk of NMS

  - lithium and sodium valproate may contribute to weight gain.

Clozapine and atypicals

- In combination with olanzapine or quetiapine may increase sedation and orthostatic hypotension.

- Amisulpride: appears to alleviate negative symptoms.

Cigarette smoking

- Shown to reduce haloperidol levels.

- Clozapine levels lowered by smoking.

- Reduces half-life of olanzapine by 21%.

- Schizophrenic cigarette smokers tend to receive higher doses of antipsychotics than non-smokers (Goff et al, 1992).

Alcohol

- Increased sedation with most antipsychotics – particularly phenothiazines, clozapine.

- Enhances sedation caused by benzodiazepines by as much as 20–30%

- *In general, assume that the effect of alcohol will be doubled in combination with antipsychotics.*

Acute situations

- Increased risk of hypotension, sedation when using IM chlorpromazine (very rare) or zuclopenthixol acetate with clozapine, olanzapine, quetiapine.

- Increased risk of sedation when using benzodiazepines with clozapine, olanzapine, quetiapine.

+ Increased risk of EPS when using haloperidol, droperidol or zuclopenthixol acetate with risperidone, amisulpride or high-dose (≥20mg) olanzapine.

Summary

Interactions occur during:

+ Acute situations

+ Chronic situations; usually treatment resistance or inadequate dosing of individual drugs

+ Affective component to psychoses

+ Cross-titrating during a switch.

Switching from one antipsychotic drug to another

Some patients may benefit by switching from a conventional to an atypical antipsychotic, from an atypical to a conventional antipsychotic, or from one atypical antipsychotic to another. Methods of switching antipsychotic therapies include tapering and cross-over strategies.

Why switch?

+ Treatment resistance

+ Treatment intolerance

+ Simplification of treatment

+ Prevention of side-effects in the future

+ Maintaining and/or enhancing adherence to medication

Treatment resistance

+ Persistence of positive symptoms

+ Persistence of negative symptoms

+ Persistence of residual symptoms at doses beyond which side-effects render treatment unacceptable.

Treatment intolerance

+ Side-effects impair quality of life

+ Side-effects can cause or add to stigma

+ Side-effects can put physical health at risk

+ Side-effects account for about 50% of non-compliance

+ Non-compliance accounts for about 80% of relapses.

Simplification of treatment

+ Especially when two or more agents are needed to address symptoms – may be more than one antipsychotic, or an antipsychotic and an anxiolytic.

+ One or more agents needed to address symptoms, and additional agents needed to address side-effects (usually antipsychotic(s) and anticholinergic medication).

+ This can be achieved by switching to an agent whose side-effects can be managed by intelligent nursing intervention rather than by adding in another drug.

Prevention of side-effects in the future

These include:

+ Tardive dyskinesia

+ Reduced fertility caused by chronic hyperprolactinaemia

+ Bone density changes caused by chronic hyperprolactinaemia.

Maintaining or enhancing adherence to medication regimens

+ Patient expresses a wish to change medication.

+ Patient finds current regimen complex and difficult to manage.

+ Patient finds side-effects or risk of developing side-effects unacceptable or incompatible with lifestyle.

+ Patient finds route of administration unacceptable (may have pain at injection sites if on depot; conversely, may prefer the simplicity of depot medication).

10 Practical guidelines for switching from one antipsychotic drug to another

To switch medication successfully it is important to:

+ Avoid relapse due to inadequate antipsychotic cover

+ Avoid withdrawal symptoms

+ Avoid confusion about new drug dosages and effects due to over-zealous cross-titration

+ Check side-effect profile of new drug, and manage accordingly

+ Adhere to principles of evidence-based practice – do pre- and post-switching rating scales

+ Check that the patient understands and is willing and able to adhere to the new treatment regimen

+ Ensure that appropriate structures are in place to support and monitor the patient during the switching period.

Specific switching strategies

From depot to oral atypical:

+ When depot is due, commence high-potency oral atypical (risperidone, olanzapine)

+ When depot is due, commence low-potency oral atypical (quetiapine, clozapine)

Opinion differs as to the 'right' time to commence oral antipsychotic therapy when switching from a depot preparation. There is evidence (Taylor, 1997b) to suggest that cross-titration is not necessary when switching from depot to oral medication.

If anticholinergics are being used, withdraw slowly to prevent:

+ Sudden appearance of EPS

+ Worsening of existing EPS

+ Worsening of tardive dyskinesia

◆ Cholinergic rebound

    – nausea

    – vomiting

    – restlessness

    – sleeplessness.

From oral conventional to atypical:

◆ Cross-titrate where possible

    – risperidone

    – olanzapine

    – quetiapine

Rationale: maintain adequate antipsychotic cover.

When switching women from a conventional neuroleptic to an atypical agent, check baseline prolactin levels, and ask about regularity and frequency of menstruation. As female patients may have experienced hyperprolactinaemia and may have been amenorrhoeic or anovulatory for some time, it is essential to warn them that they will probably start menstruating again and that fertility may return to pre-treatment levels within the next few months. Advice about, or access to advice about family planning and methods of contraception should always be offered. If a patient has been hyperprolactinaemic, it is likely that her libido has also been low – it is worth reminding patients that this will probably return to normal within the next 6–8 weeks. Recheck prolactin levels in 6 weeks, and if still raised, recheck in 3 months. If menstruation (in women of child-bearing age) has not returned to normal within 6 months, refer to specialist gynaecology/endocrinology clinic.

Patients may retain symptoms of hyperprolactinaemia for some months although prolactin levels have returned to normal.

When starting clozapine

- Withdraw oral conventional agent first to reduce possibility of:

  – Neutropenia

  – Lowered seizure threshold

- If in doubt about adequate antipsychotic cover, either:

  – Cross-titrate – after analysing risk of relapse vs risk of neutropenia/seizure

  – Admit to hospital for duration of switch

  – Add benzodiazepine

Switching from one atypical to another

- Avoid abrupt clozapine withdrawal (not usually possible – patients normally stop clozapine treatment either because of neutropenia, where a sudden cessation of treatment is necessary to minimize physical risk, or because of non-compliance)

- Avoid abrupt withdrawal of atypical antipsychotics to avoid rebound psychosis

- Cross-titrate where possible

- Where switching from low-potency antipsychotic, maintain adequate anticholinergic cover to avoid cholinergic rebound

Reasons for not switching

- Patient expresses a wish to remain on current medication

- Compliance may be impaired

- No need: stable, no side-effects

Investing in the future

- Better quality of life – atypical antipsychotic drugs are as effective against positive symptoms, potentially more effective against negative symptoms

- Improved compliance – a more tolerable and manageable side-effect profile

- Minimizing the risk of tardive dyskinesia

- Minimizing cognitive impairment

- Cost of drugs is only 3% of total cost of schizophrenia (Byrom et al, 1998)

11 Scenarios for switching: sample case vignettes

Case study I

Steven B, a 30-year-old man with a 12-year history of schizophrenia, has been taking depot flupenthixol for the past 6 years. His current dose is 200mg/2-weekly. Prior to that, he was on fluphenazine decanoate. His positive symptoms (command auditory hallucinations, paranoid delusions of being followed) have remained fairly well controlled on this regimen. However, he is socially withdrawn, and spends most of his time lying on his bed or watching television in his room. His self-care is generally poor.

He also suffers from akathisia, and stiffness in his limbs. A rating scale assessment gave a score of 10 on the Simpson–Angus scale (score range 0–36) and 6 on the Barnes akathisia scale (score range 0–14). He has always been poorly compliant, although has never actually refused medication. When reminded to attend for depot injections, he has always done so. He is currently in warden-controlled accommodation, and has a supportive CPN.

Switch to:

+ Oral atypical – probably not quetiapine, because of bd dosage. Clozapine not indicated at this stage.

+ Start olanzapine or risperidone at the end of the depot cycle.

+ Slowly withdraw procyclidine over 2–3 months to avoid cholinergic rebound.

+ Compliance therapy.

+ Enlist the aid of warden to remind him to take medication.

+ Provide a dosette box.

Factors to consider:

+ Possibility of this man developing tardive dyskinesia.

+ Akathisia implicated in suicide in schizophrenia (est. 40%) (Levine, 1999).

+ Withdraw procyclidine slowly.

+ Address negative symptoms.

+ Importance of psychosocial interventions.

◆   If commencing olanzapine, ensure patient receives pre-treatment weight management counselling – refer to dietician or weight clinic.

Case study II

Anna F is a 71-year-old woman who was admitted to hospital after being brought to the emergency clinic by her daughter. Anna's neighbour had telephoned the daughter when she became concerned at Anna's 'strange behaviour', which included going through the rubbish bins at night, locking herself in her flat and refusing to answer the neighbour's knocks on the door, and repeatedly shouting 'Get out! Get out!' at frequent intervals through the night when there was nobody else in the flat. When her daughter arrived, Anna told her that the secret service had sent spies into the flat, and that she had been trying to find them.

She was diagnosed as having paraphrenia, and commenced on haloperidol 3mg bd. Anna's symptoms improved, but on visiting her in hospital her daughter was horrified to find her looking like a 'zombie', with a stiff gait, mask-like face and a tremor. She demanded that something be done about the medication, and it was agreed that something would be done.

Switch to:

◆   Low D2 blocker, as patient is sensitive to haloperidol.

◆   Quetiapine a good choice for elderly patients as it is mildly sedating, rarely causes EPS and is well-tolerated across a wide dose spectrum.

◆   Commence starter pack – in elderly patients, starter pack may need to be given over 8 days, using once daily.

Factors to consider:

◆   Orthostatic hypotension may have serious consequences (falls, fractures).

◆   Patient's age and associated risks – falls, tremor and possibility of accidents.

◆   Choose a drug offering a broad dose spectrum with a wide therapeutic window.

Case study III

Helen S, a 38-year-old woman, has been treated successfully with clozapine 500mg for > 6 years. She had previously been treatment resistant – conventional neuroleptics had failed to give any relief from her constant auditory hallucinations. While on clozapine she gained some weight, but was unconcerned about this and remained within a healthy weight range. Unfortunately, Helen developed neutropenia, and was given a 'red alert' by the clozapine monitoring service. She has had to stop taking clozapine.

Switch to:

✦ Oral atypical – olanzapine, quetiapine, risperidone or amisulpride.

✦ If ineffective at therapeutic dose ranges, consider increasing slightly.

✦ Consider adding low dose of benzodiazepine short-term while starting a cognitive intervention to help her cope with any hallucinations.

✦ If still no relief, restart clozapine if permitted as soon as it is safe to do so. (This will need to be negotiated with the Clozaril Patient Monitoring Service.)

Factors to consider:*

✦ Abrupt withdrawal of clozapine necessary here. Watch for rebound psychosis and cholinergic rebound.

✦ Patient should probably be hospitalized if practical.

✦ Consider anticholinergic cover or short-term benzodiazepine cover.

✦ Weight gain not an issue here, but continue to monitor weight.

* Clozapine-induced neutropenia usually occurs during the first 18 weeks of treatment, and by the end of the first year at the latest. 'Coincidental' neutropenia may occur at any time – is often a 'rogue' low result, or a normal finding in black patients caused by an artefact (white cell aggregation at the sides of the blood collection tube).

Case study IV

Sophie B is a 29-year-old woman who was first diagnosed as having schizophrenia 8 years ago. She was treated unsuccessfully for 7 years with a variety of neuroleptics – chlorpromazine, zuclopenthixol and sulpiride – before her team decided to try and treat her illness with an atypical agent. While on conventional neuroleptics, her symptoms – distressing auditory hallucinations telling her she was evil and deserved to die – never fully abated, and she had actually made two serious suicide attempts. She also suffered from quite severe negative symptoms, being withdrawn, apathetic and amotivated, with poor self-care and social skills, despite neuropsychological tests that showed her to be of above average intelligence.

A trial of olanzapine afforded some improvement in her negative symptoms, but failed to effect any change in her psychotic symptomatology. What would you suggest as the most appropriate treatment for this patient, and why? She is currently taking olanzapine 20mg/day.

Switch to:

- Clozapine, as unlikely another atypical will be any more successful than olanzapine in treating positive symptoms.

- If patient unwilling to try clozapine, try another atypical and add an antidepressant.

Factors to consider:

- Patient will require careful monitoring during switching period – may be a high suicide risk.

- Clozapine helpful in preventing suicide (Meltzer and Okayli, 1995).

- Pre-and post-treatment weight counselling.

- Record baseline weight, blood glucose levels and triglycerides.

- Consider CBT to help with any residual psychotic symptoms.

Case study V

> Gordon S is a 38-year-old man who tried to kill his wife 2 years ago because he thought she was possessed by the devil. He has a long history of paranoid schizophrenia, and although his symptoms have been well controlled on depot flupenthixol, he has developed tardive dyskinesia. He is angry about this, and although very remorseful about what he did to his wife, he has become poorly compliant and is in danger of relapsing and being recalled to hospital for a very long admission. He is currently living in supervised accommodation.
>
> His consultant feels strongly that Gordon has a right to the best possible treatment and would like to switch him to an oral atypical, but is naturally worried that Gordon may not comply with his new medication regimen.

Switch to:

- Atypical with low D2 blockade. Clozapine not indicated at this stage.

- Olanzapine or quetiapine as the drug of choice: both low D2 blockade (at ≥20mg for olanzapine). If not responding to 15mg olanzapine, consider switching to quetiapine or clozapine. Raising the dose of olanzapine beyond 15mg will result in higher levels of D2 blockade, increasing the risk of EPS in a patient known to be sensitive to this problem (Kapur et al, 2000a).

- Rationale for these choices is that both drugs have assays for checking compliance.

- As compliance is vital, olanzapine may be the drug of choice as it only requires once-daily dosage.

+ Clozapine and quetiapine both known to have been effective in reversing tardive dyskinesia.

Factors to consider:

+ Pre-treatment weight counselling if starting olanzapine.

+ Baseline weight, glucose and cholesterol, LFTs.

+ Patient may need higher dose of olanzapine if a smoker.

+ Patient should have regular drug plasma levels to check compliance.

+ If in supervised accommodation, enlist aid of staff to help supervise medication.

Case study VI

John D, a 45-year-old man, has been treated with zuclopenthixol 200mg/2-weekly for the past 15 years. His positive symptoms have responded well, but he is socially withdrawn and shows little interest in his surroundings. He has attended a day centre for some years, but has not formed any relationships with other patients and often declines to join in activities, preferring to sit alone. He denies depression and scored 0 on the Calgary Depression Scale. His psychiatrist feels that he may respond well to an oral atypical agent, and has sent John for review. John is very happy to continue taking his depot, and denies any side-effects. Of his social isolation, he claims to have always preferred his own company, and says he has never needed friends. He said he would probably get confused with tablets, and that the fortnightly visits to the depot clinic fit in well with his lifestyle.

Switch to:

+ A switch is not indicated in this case for several reasons:

  – Patient is happy with his medication

  – Patient does not appear to be suffering from side-effects

  – Patient's social withdrawal is probably not due to negative symptoms

  – Patient has expressed doubts about ability to comply with oral medication.

Factors to consider:

+ Patient may develop side-effects in the future and should be regularly monitored.

+ If patient does switch to an oral medication, he will need support with adhering to the regimen.

Case study VII

Robert A, a 26-year-old man, was diagnosed with paranoid schizophrenia 3 years ago. He was prescribed depot haloperidol, but remained psychotic for some months. When his dose of depot was increased, he developed severe dystonia. He was switched to risperidone 6 months ago, and has responded very well. He is currently taking 6mg/day. However, he is still suffering from mild dystonia and has also developed erectile dysfunction. This is bothering him as he has recently started a relationship. A recent prolactin level was high (735mmol/l). He is unwilling to change medication as he says it is such a relief to be well again.

Switch to:

✦ Switch not indicated at this stage. Reduce risperidone gradually by 1mg/week and monitor symptoms and side-effects (using rating scales) carefully. If symptoms reappear, increase dose by 1mg, and then try reducing by 0.5mg.

✦ If psychiatric symptoms reappear when patient is still experiencing sexual problems, consider switching to a low D2 blocker such as quetiapine or olanzapine.

Factors to consider:

✦ Continue to monitor prolactin levels while dose of risperidone is reduced.

✦ Dystonia may still be a residual effect of depot.

✦ If sexual problems persist after prolactin levels return to normal, consider referral to a sexual health clinic.

✦ Inform patient that sexual function may not improve for 6–8 weeks after changes in medication are instituted and prolactin levels have returned to normal.

✦ In normoprolactinaemic men, autonomic side-effects are the primary cause of sexual dysfunction and hyperprolactinaemia overrides other antipsychotic-induced sexual dysfunctions.

12 Guide to collecting and interpreting atypical antipsychotic plasma levels

Drug	Level available	Method of collection	Target range
Clozapine	Yes	Plasma >2.5ml EDTA tube	Clozapine 350–700µg/l
			Norclozapine >45µg/l
Olanzapine	Yes	Plasma >5ml EDTA tube	Trough: >9mg/l 12hrs post: >23mg/l >40mg/l probably unnecessary for therapeutic effect
Quetiapine	Yes	Plasma >5ml EDTA tube or serum >2ml	No therapeutic target range – measured levels vary from 20 to 500µg/l
Risperidone*	No	x	No therapeutic range available as yet
Amisulpride	Yes	Plasma >5ml plain tube (gel)	No therapeutic target range available as yet

*Risperidone can be detected in the blood. However, as yet there is no available assay for therapeutic range. Defecting the presence of the drug may be a useful tool in determining compliance.

Guidelines for collecting blood levels

Patient must consent to blood level being taken, and understand the procedure and the implications of the procedure.

When requesting a blood level analysis, it is essential to record the following information on the request form:

✦ Dose of medication

✦ Usual times of administration

✦ Time last dose was taken and dose in milligrams

✦ Any other current medication

✦ Weight of patient (if known)

✦ If on clozapine or olanzapine, whether patient is a smoker

✦ Whether any physical condition may be affecting level (e.g. diarrhoea/vomiting).

13 Managing side-effects

> ✦ A side-effect is an effect (usually for the worse) of a drug other than that for which it is administered *(Shorter Oxford Dictionary)*

Why do we see such big variations in side-effects between different antipsychotic agents?

> ✦ Different receptor binding profiles
>
> ✦ Extent and site of D2 blockade is the main difference between the 'typicals' and the 'atypicals'
>
> ✦ An 'atypical' drug is one that does not cause EPS at clinically effective doses

Effects of D2 blockade

Location	Effect
Striatum	Extrapyramidal side-effects
Hypothalamus	Hyperprolactinaemia
Cerebral cortex	Antipsychotic action Suggested reduction in negative symptoms

Variations in receptor binding profiles

Receptor	Low-potency typical	Haloperidol	Risperidone	Olanzapine	Quetiapine	Amisulpride	Clozapine
D2	Yes	Yes	Yes	Yes	Yes	Yes	Yes
D3	No	No	No	Yes	No	Yes	Yes
5HT	Yes	No	Yes	Yes	Yes	No	Yes
M	Yes	No	No	Yes	No	No	Yes
H	Yes	No	No	Yes	Yes	No	Yes
α	Yes	Yes	Yes	Yes	Yes	No	Yes

D, dopamine; 5HT, serotonin; M, muscarinic; H, histamine; A, adrinergic.

Other reasons for variance in side-effects are:

✦   Idiosyncratic reactions among individual patients

✦   Effects of other drugs, e.g. nicotine, caffeine

✦   Side-effects may be dose-related, and dissipate when dose is reduced.

Consequences of side-effects

Psychological, social
Physical
Often a combination of the above – a cause and effect relationship

Non-compliance

✦   Devastating in its effect on outcome

One of the main reasons for non-compliance is side-effects (Nasrallah and Mulvihill, 2001).

✦   >95% of first-onset presentations relapsed within 5 years of stopping medication (Robinson et al, 1999).

Psychosocial effects of side-effects

+   Non-compliance and consequent relapse or inadequate control of symptoms

+   Stigma and social isolation due to 'odd' appearance

+   Impaired quality of life

+   Depression: due to existence of side-effects or secondary to D2 blockade

+   Suicide: estimated 40% due to akathisia (Levine, 1998)

Variations in side-effects

Side effect	Low-potency typical	Haloperidol	Risperidone	Olanzapine	Quetiapine	Amisulpride	Clozapine
EPS	Yes	Yes	Yes*	Rare**	No	Yes	No
Sedation	Varies	No	No	Yes	Yes	No	Yes
Weight gain	Yes + - ++	Yes +	Yes +	Yes ++	Yes +	Yes +	Yes ++
Anti-cholinergic	Varies	No	No	Yes	No	No	Yes
Raised prolactin	Yes	Yes	Yes*	Rare*	No	Yes	No

* Dose-related: some women may experience symptomatic hyperprolactinaemia and EPS at doses as low as 2mg risperidone, men at higher doses. ** Patients rarely experience hyperprolactinaemia or EPS at doses of <20mg/day olanzapine.

The most common physical side-effects likely to be experienced are:

+   Acute dystonia, discomfort, pain

+   Parkinsonism – discomfort, pain, dysthymia

+   Akathisia – discomfort, pain, dysthymia

+   Tardive dyskinesia – stigmatizing

+   Sedation, lethargy

- Orthostatic hypotension: dizziness, falls

- Anticholinergic effects: dry mouth, constipation, bowel obstruction

- Lowered seizure threshold: fits, or more drugs

- Hyperprolactinaemia: lowered libido, impotence, amenorrhoea, risk of reduced fertility, increased risk of osteoporosis

- Weight gain: increased risk of heart disease, hypertension, type II diabetes, cancer

- Cardiovascular effects – prolonged QTc interval

- Agitation, anxiety

- Neuroleptic malignant syndrome (NMS)

- Myocarditis

- Neutropenia which may progress to agranulocytosis (as about 4% of patients on clozapine experience blood dyscrasias, all patients receiving clozapine require regular blood monitoring)

- Nausea, vomiting, gastric reflux

- Photosensitivity.

Balancing risks of inadequately treated mental illness against the risks of side-effects

- The differences between newer (atypical) agents (in their propensity to cause weight gain) may influence compliance and health risk (Allison et al, 1999)

- 492 suicides per 100,000 over 10 years prevented by clozapine

- 416 deaths per 100,000 over 10 years due to antipsychotic-induced weight gain

- 'Results suggest that lives saved by clozapine may essentially be offset by deaths due to weight gain' (Fontaine et al, 2001)

Identifying side-effects

- Requires awareness of individual drug neuropharmacology and likely side-effects

- Asking the patient, particularly about sensitive issues such as sexual function, which the patient may not feel comfortable about mentioning him/herself

- Use of rating scales – LUNSERS, AIMS, Barnes, Simpson–Angus, Schizophrenia Quality of Life Scale

- Regular weight checks, glucose tolerance tests if at risk

Management of side-effects

- Side-effects of typicals usually require drug (anticholinergic) intervention.

- Side-effects of atypicals can, on the whole, be managed by intelligent nursing intervention.

Sedation

- Usually transient

- Usually more manageable if the patient is forewarned

- Can often be alleviated by changing dosing schedule

- Can often be alleviated by behavioural goal-setting techniques

- May require reduction in dose or, in extreme cases, changing to another drug

Orthostatic hypotension

- Usually transient
- Can usually be managed by nursing advice such as:
  - Not getting up from lying or sitting position too quickly
  - Not getting out of a hot bath quickly
- May be dose related
- May improve by switching from a low-potency drug to a high-potency drug

Anticholinergic effects

- Constipation: water, exercise, roughage
- Dry mouth: water, sugar-free sweets or chewing gum
- Sialorrhoea (drooling) (clozapine): sleeping on an extra pillow, placing a towel on pillow; in extreme cases may require treatment with hyoscine or pirenzepine

Weight gain

- Pre-treatment planning is the ideal
- Referral to dietician or other weight clinic
- Advice on healthy eating and exercise
- Enlist the aid of carers, other involved professionals
- Motivational interviewing, realistic goal-setting
- Education about potential consequences of obesity
- In extreme cases, change medication or consider adding a weight loss agent
- Baseline and regular weight, glucose tolerance and triglyceride level testing

Hyperprolactinaemia and EPS in atypicals

- ✦ Usually dose related

- ✦ Check serum prolactin/pregnancy test

- ✦ Reduce dose until side-effects no longer present

- ✦ If clinical effect is not achieved at this dose, consider changing medication after consulting patient

---

Some side-effects – if distressing or injurious to health – may require switching to an alternative agent. These include:

- ✦ NMS

- ✦ Neutropenia/agranulocytosis

- ✦ Myocarditis

- ✦ Cardiac rhythm abnormalities

- ✦ Impaired glucose tolerance

Prevention is better than cure:

- ✦ Keep patients informed

- ✦ Keep carers informed

- ✦ Regular contact and encouragement in early stages

- ✦ Baseline and regular side-effect scales, quality of life scales, symptom rating scales.

Summary

✦   Side-effects are generated by the pharmacological action of the drug

✦   Some are more tolerable than others

✦   Some have very serious consequences

✦   Nurses can identify and manage most side-effects generated by atypical medications by using a holistic, patient-centred approach

✦   Prevention is better than cure

✦   Optimum quality of life and cost-effectiveness can be achieved by switching to an agent whereby side-effects can be managed by intelligent nursing intervention rather than by adding in another drug.

Appendix I: Normal blood values

Blood biochemistry: normal values

	SI units	Conventional units
Acid–base measurement		
Base excess	+/– 2mmol/l	+/– 2mEq/l
Bicarbonate	24–33mmol/l	24/33mEq/l
Arterial:		
H^+ concentration (pH)	36–45µmol/l	pH 7.37–7.45
pCO_2	4.5–6.1kPa	35–46mmHg
pCO_2	12–15kPa	90–110mmHg
Electrolytes		
Calcium	2.1–2.8mmol/l	8.5–10.5mg/100ml
Chloride	96–108mmol/l	96–108mEq/l
Phosphate (as inorganic P)	0.65–1.62mol/l	2.0–5.0mg/100ml
Potassium	3.5–5.5mmol/l	3.5–5.5mEq/l
Sodium	135–145mmol/l	135–145mEq/l
Proteins		
Total proteins	62–82g/l	6.2–8.2g/100ml
Albumin	36–52g/l	3.6–5.2g/100ml
Globulin	24–37g/l	2.4–3.7g/100ml
Liver function		
Alanine aminotransferase (ALAT)	10–40U/l	
Albumin	36–62g/l	3.6–5.2g/100ml
Alkaline phosphatase	30–92U/l	3.0–13.0KA units
Aspartate aminotransferase (ASAT)	10–40 units	
Bilirubin (total)	2–17µmol/l	0.2–1.0mg/100ml
Globulin	24–37g/l	2.4–3.7g/100ml

Lactate dehydrogenase (LDH)	100–300U/l	
Others		
Acid phosphatase	0.1–0.4U/l	0.5–5.0KA units
Amylase	50–300 units	
Creatinine	60–120µmol/l	0.7–1.4mg/100ml
Creatinine clearance	97–127ml/min	
Glucose (fasting)	3.3–6.7mmol/l	60–100mg/100ml
Hydroxybutyrate dehydrogenase (HBD)	70–190U/l	
Iron	11–32µmol/l	60–180µg/100ml
Iron binding capacity	45–70µmol/l	250–400µg/100ml
Lead	0.5–2.0µmol/l	10–40µg/100ml
Protein-bound iodine (PBI)	300–600nmol/l	4.0–7.5µg/100ml
Triglycerides	0.83–1.92mmol/l	74–172mg/100ml
Urate	0.1–0.4mmol/l	2.0–7.0mg/100ml
Urea	1.7–7.5mmol/l	10–45mg/100ml

Blood haematology: normal values

Red cells – erythrocytes		
Red cell count (RBC)	Male	4.6–6.2 million/mm^3
	Female	4.2–5.4 million/mm^3
Reticulocytes		<2% of red cells
Haemoglobin	Male	14–18g/100ml
	Female	12–16g/100ml
PCV haematocrit	Male	40–54g/100ml
	Female	37–47g/100ml
MCV (mean corpuscular volume)		73.5–98.7µm^3

MCHC (mean corpuscular haemoglobin concentration)		31.3–36.9g/100ml
ESR (erythrocyte sedimentation rate)	Male	0–9mm/h (Wintrobe)
		1–5mm/h (Westergren)
	Female	0–15mm/h (Wintrobe)
		4–7mm/h (Westergren)
White cells – leukocytes		
Total white cell count		$4.8–10.8 \times 10^9/l$
Neutrophils		$2.5–7.5 \times 10^9/l$
Lymphocytes		$1.0–4.5 \times 10^9/l$
Eosinophils		$0.05–0.4 \times 10^9/l$
Basophils		$0–0.2 \times 10^9/l$
Monocytes		$0.2–0.9 \times 10^9/l$
Thrombocytes (platelets)		$150–400 \times 10^9/l$
Blood coagulation		
Bleeding time		2.5–7min (Ivy)
Coagulation time (capillary)		5–7min (Wright)
Coagulation time (venous)		4–7min (Lee & White)
Prothrombin time		10–14s (Quick)
Prolactin (different laboratories may have different reference ranges)	Male	<550 mU/l
	Female	<650 mU/l

Appendix II: Rating scales

The following scales appear in this section:

+ PANSS (Positive and Negative Symptom Scale)

+ BPRS (Brief Psychiatric Rating Scale)

+ CGI (Clinical Global Impression)

+ GAS (Global Assessment Scale)

+ HONOS (Health of the Nation Outcome Scale)

+ Calgary Depression Scale

+ Schizophrenia Quality of Life Scale

+ Simpson–Angus Scale

+ Barnes Akathisia Scale

+ AIMS (Abnormal Involuntary Movements Scale)

+ LUNSERS (Liverpool University Side-effects Rating Scale)

+ SFQ (Sexual Functioning Questionnaire)

+ Sexual Dysfunction Checklist

+ Client Service Receipt Inventory

+ DAI-10 (Drug Attitude Inventory)

+ UKU Side-effects Scale

PANSS (Positive and Negative Symptoms Scale)

POSITIVE SCALE (P)

(Tick one box only for each assessment)

P1. Delusions. Beliefs which are unfounded, unrealistic, and idiosyncratic. **Basis for rating:** thought content expressed in the interview and its influence on social relations and behaviour.

- ☐ 1 **Absent** – Definition does not apply.
- ☐ 2 **Minimal** – Questionable pathology; may be at the upper extreme of normal limits.
- ☐ 3 **Mild** – Presence of one or two delusions which are vague, uncrystallised, and not tenaciously held. Delusions do not interfere with thinking, social relations, or behaviour.
- ☐ 4 **Moderate** – Presence of either a kaleidoscopic array of poorly formed, unstable delusions or of a few well-formed delusions that occasionally interfere with thinking, social relations, or behaviour.
- ☐ 5 **Moderate severe** – Presence of numerous well-formed delusions that are tenaciously held and occasionally interfere with thinking, social relations, or behaviour.
- ☐ 6 **Severe** – Presence of a stable set of delusions which are crystallised, possibly systematised, tenaciously held, and clearly interfere with thinking, social relations, and behaviour.
- ☐ 7 **Extreme** – Presence of a stable set of delusions which are either highly systematised or very
- 3 numerous, and which dominate major facets of the patient's life. This frequently results in inappropriate and irresponsible action, which may even jeopardise the safety of the patient or others.

P2. Conceptual disorganisation. Disorganised process of thinking characterised by disruption of goal-directed sequencing, e.g. circumstantiality, tangentiality, loose associations, non sequiturs, gross illogicality, or thought block. **Basis for rating:** cognitive-verbal processes observed during the course of the interview.

- ☐ 1 **Absent** – Definition does not apply.
- ☐ 2 **Minimal** – Questionable pathology; may be at the upper extreme of normal limits.
- ☐ 3 **Mild** – Thinking is circumstantial, tangential, or paralogical. There is some difficulty in directing thoughts toward a goal, and some loosening of associations may be evidenced under pressure.
- ☐ 4 **Moderate** – Able to focus thoughts when communications are brief and structured, but becomes loose or irrelevant when dealing with more complex communications or when under minimal pressure.
- ☐ 5 **Moderate severe** – Generally has difficulty in organising thoughts, as evidenced by frequent irrelevancies, disconnectedness, or loosening of associations even when not under pressure.
- ☐ 6 **Severe** – Thinking is seriously derailed and internally inconsistent, resulting in gross irrelevancies and disruption of thought processes, which occur almost constantly.
- ☐ 7 **Extreme** – Thoughts are disrupted to the point where the patient is incoherent. There is
- 4 marked loosening of associations, which results in total failure of communication, e.g. 'word salad' or mutism.

P3. Hallucinatory behaviour. Verbal report or behaviour indicating perceptions which are not generated by external stimuli. These may occur in the auditory, visual, olfactory, or somatic realms. **Basis for rating:** verbal report and physical manifestations during the course of interview as well as reports of behaviour by primary care workers or family.

- ☐ 1 **Absent** – Definition does not apply.
- ☐ 2 **Minimal** – Questionable pathology; may be at the upper extreme of normal limits.
- ☐ 3 **Mild** – One or two clearly formed but infrequent hallucinations, or else a number of vague abnormal perceptions which do not result in distortions of thinking or behaviour.
- ☐ 4 **Moderate** – Hallucinations occur frequently but not continuously, and the patient's thinking and behaviour are affected only to a minor extent.
- ☐ 5 **Moderate severe** – Hallucinations are frequent, may involve more than one sensory modality, and tend to distort thinking and/or disrupt behaviour. Patient may have delusional interpretation of these experiences and respond to them emotionally and, on occasion, verbally as well.
- ☐ 6 **Severe** – Hallucinations are present almost continuously, causing major disruption of thinking and behaviour. Patient treats these as real perceptions, and functioning is impeded by frequent emotional and verbal responses to them.
- ☐ 7 **Extreme** – Patient is almost totally preoccupied with hallucinations, which virtually
- 5   dominate thinking and behaviour. Hallucinations are provided a rigid delusional interpretation and provoke verbal and behavioural responses, including obedience to command hallucinations.

P4. Excitement. Hyperactivity as reflected in accelerated motor behaviour, heightened responsivity to stimuli, hypervigilance, or excessive mood lability. **Basis for rating:** behavioural manifestations during the course of interview as well as reports of behaviour by primary care workers or family.

- ☐ 1 **Absent** – Definition does not apply.
- ☐ 2 **Minimal** – Questionable pathology; may be at the upper extreme of normal limits.
- ☐ 3 **Mild** – Tends to be slightly agitated, hypervigilant, or mildly overaroused throughout the interview, but without distinct episodes of excitement or marked mood lability. Speech may be slightly pressured.
- ☐ 4 **Moderate** – Agitation or overarousal is clearly evident throughout the interview, affecting speech and general mobility, or episodic outbursts occur sporadically.
- ☐ 5 **Moderate severe** – Significant hyperactivity or frequent outbursts of motor activity are observed, making it difficult for the patient to sit still for longer than several minutes at any given time.
- ☐ 6 **Severe** – Marked excitement dominates the interview, delimits attention, and to some extent affects personal functions such as eating and sleeping.
- ☐ 7 **Extreme** – Marked excitement seriously interferes in eating and sleeping and makes
- 6   interpersonal interactions virtually impossible. Acceleration of speech and motor activity may result in incoherence and exhaustion.

P5. Grandiosity. Exaggerated self-opinion and unrealistic convictions of superiority, including delusions of extraordinary abilities, wealth, knowledge, fame, power, and moral righteousness. **Basis for rating:** thought content expressed in the interview and its influence on behaviour.

- ☐ 1 **Absent** – Definition does not apply.
- ☐ 2 **Minimal** – Questionable pathology; may be at the upper extreme of normal limits.
- ☐ 3 **Mild** – Some expansiveness or boastfulness is evident, but without clear-cut grandiose delusions.
- ☐ 4 **Moderate** – Feels distinctly and unrealistically superior to others. Some poorly formed delusions about special status or abilities may be present but are not acted upon.
- ☐ 5 **Moderate severe** – Clear-cut delusions concerning remarkable abilities, status, or power are expressed and influence attitude but not behaviour.
- ☐ 6 **Severe** – Clear-cut delusions of remarkable superiority involving more than one parameter (wealth, knowledge, fame, etc.) are expressed, notably influence interactions, and may be acted upon.
- ☐ 7 **Extreme** – Thinking, interactions, and behaviour are dominated by multiple delusions of
- 7 amazing ability, wealth, knowledge, fame, power, and/or moral stature, which may take on a bizarre quality.

P6. Suspiciousness/persecution. Unrealistic or exaggerated ideas of persecution, as reflected in guardedness, a distrustful attitude, suspicious hypervigilance, or frank delusions that others mean one harm. **Basis for rating:** thought content expressed in the interview and its influence on behaviour.

- ☐ 1 **Absent** – Definition does not apply.
- ☐ 2 **Minimal** – Questionable pathology; may be at the upper extreme of normal limits.
- ☐ 3 **Mild** – Presents a guarded or even openly distrustful attitude, but thoughts, interactions, and behaviour are minimally affected.
- ☐ 4 **Moderate** – Distrustfulness is clearly evident and intrudes on the interview and/or behaviour, but there is no evidence of persecutory delusions. Alternatively, there may be indication of loosely formed persecutory delusions, but these do not seem to affect the patient's attitude or interpersonal relations.
- ☐ 5 **Moderate severe** – Patient shows marked distrustfulness, leading to major disruption of interpersonal relations, or else there are clear-cut persecutory delusions that have limited impact on interpersonal relations and behaviour.
- ☐ 6 **Severe** – Clear-cut pervasive delusions of persecution which may be systematised and significantly interfere in interpersonal relations.
- ☐ 7 **Extreme** – A network of systematised persecutory delusions dominates the patient's
- 8 thinking, social relations, and behaviour.

P7. Hostility. Verbal and nonverbal expressions of anger and resentment, including sarcasm, passive-aggressive behaviour, verbal abuse, and assaultiveness. **Basis for rating:** interpersonal behaviour observed during the interview and reports by primary care workers or family.

- ☐ 1 **Absent** – Definition does not apply.
- ☐ 2 **Minimal** – Questionable pathology; may be at the upper extreme of normal limits.
- ☐ 3 **Mild** – Indirect or restrained communication of anger, such as sarcasm, disrespect, hostile expressions, and occasional irritability.
- ☐ 4 **Moderate** – Presents an overtly hostile attitude, showing frequent irritability and direct expression of anger or resentment.
- ☐ 5 **Moderate severe** – Patient is highly irritable and occasionally verbally abusive or threatening.
- ☐ 6 **Severe** – Uncooperativeness and verbal abuse or threats notably influence the interview and seriously impact upon social relations. Patient may be violent and destructive but is not physically assaultive toward others.
- ☐ 7 **Extreme** – Marked anger results in extreme uncooperativeness, precluding other
- 9 interactions, or in episode(s) of physical assault toward others.

NEGATIVE SCALE (N)

N1. Blunted affect. Diminished emotional responsiveness as characterised by a reduction in facial expression, modulation of feelings, and communicative gestures. **Basis for rating:** observation of physical manifestations of affective tone and emotional responsiveness during the course of the interview.

- ☐ 1 **Absent** – Definition does not apply.
- ☐ 2 **Minimal** – Questionable pathology; may be at the upper extreme of normal limits.
- ☐ 3 **Mild** – Changes in facial expression and communicative gestures seem to be stilted, forced, artificial, or lacking in modulation.
- ☐ 4 **Moderate** – Reduced range of facial expression and few expressive gestures result in a dull appearance.
- ☐ 5 **Moderate severe** – Affect is generally 'flat', with only occasional changes in facial expression and a paucity of communicative gestures.
- ☐ 6 **Severe** – Marked flatness and deficiency of emotions exhibited most of the time. There may be unmodulated extreme affective discharges, such as excitement, rage, or inappropriate uncontrolled laughter.
- ☐ 7 **Extreme** – Changes in facial expression and evidence of communicative gestures are
- 10 virtually absent. Patient seems constantly to show a barren or 'wooden' expression.

N2. Emotional withdrawal. Lack of interest in, involvement with, and affective commitment to life's events. **Basis for rating:** reports of functioning form primary care workers or family and observation of interpersonal behaviour during the course of the interview.

- ☐ 1 **Absent** – Definition does not apply.
- ☐ 2 **Minimal** – Questionable pathology; may be at the upper extreme of normal limits.
- ☐ 3 **Mild** – Usually lacks initiative and occasionally may show deficient interest in surrounding events.
- ☐ 4 **Moderate** – Patient is generally distanced emotionally from the milieu and its challenges but, with encouragement, can be engaged.
- ☐ 5 **Moderate severe** – Patient is clearly detached emotionally from persons and events in the milieu, resisting all efforts at engagement. Patient appears distant, docile, and purposeless but can be involved in communication at least briefly and tends to personal needs, sometimes with assistance.
- ☐ 6 **Severe** – Marked deficiency of interest and emotional commitment results in limited conversation with others and frequent neglect of personal functions, for which the patient requires supervision.
- ☐ 7 **Extreme** – Patient is almost totally withdrawn, uncommunicative, and neglectful of
- 11   personal needs as a result of profound lack of interest and emotional commitment.

N3. Poor rapport. Lack of interpersonal empathy, openness in conversation, and sense of closeness, interest, or involvement with the interviewer. This is evidenced by interpersonal distancing and reduced verbal and nonverbal communication. **Basis for rating:** interpersonal behaviour during the course of the interview.

- ☐ 1 **Absent** – Definition does not apply.
- ☐ 2 **Minimal** – Questionable pathology; may be at the upper extreme of normal limits.
- ☐ 3 **Mild** – Conversation is characterised by a stilted, strained, or artificial tone. It may lack emotional depth or tend to remain on an impersonal, intellectual plane.
- ☐ 4 **Moderate** – Patient typically is aloof, with interpersonal distance quite evident. Patient may answer questions mechanically, act bored, or express disinterest.
- ☐ 5 **Moderate severe** – Disinvolvement is obvious and clearly impedes the productivity of the interview. Patient may tend to avoid eye or face contact.
- ☐ 6 **Severe** – Patient is highly indifferent, with marked interpersonal distance. Answers are perfunctory, and there is little nonverbal evidence of involvement. Eye and face contact are frequently avoided.
- ☐ 7 **Extreme** – Patient is totally uninvolved with the interviewer. Patient appears to be
- 12   completely indifferent and consistently avoids verbal and nonverbal interactions during the interview.

N4. Passive/apathetic social withdrawal. Diminished interest and initiative in social interactions due to passivity, apathy, anergy, or avolition. This leads to reduced interpersonal involvements and neglect of activities of daily living. **Basis for rating:** reports on social behaviour from primary care workers or family.

- ☐ 1   **Absent** – Definition does not apply.
- ☐ 2   **Minimal** – Questionable pathology; may be at the upper extreme of normal limits.
- ☐ 3   **Mild** – Shows occasional interest in social activities but poor initiative. Usually engages with others only when approached first by them.
- ☐ 4   **Moderate** – Passively goes along with most social activities but in a disinterested or mechanical way. Tends to recede into the background.
- ☐ 5   **Moderate severe** – Passively participates in only a minority of activities and shows virtually no interest or initiative. Generally spends little time with others.
- ☐ 6   **Severe** – Tends to be apathetic and isolated, participating very rarely in social activities and occasionally neglecting personal needs. Has very few spontaneous social contacts.
- ☐ 7   **Extreme** – Profoundly apathetic, socially isolated, and personally neglectful.

13

N5. Difficulty in abstract thinking. Impairment in the use of the abstract-symbolic mode of thinking, as evidenced by difficulty in classification, forming generalisations, and proceeding beyond concrete or egocentric thinking in problem-solving tasks. **Basis for rating:** responses to questions on similarities and proverb interpretation, and use of concrete vs. abstract mode during the course of the interview.

- ☐ 1   **Absent** – Definition does not apply.
- ☐ 2   **Minimal** – Questionable pathology; may be at the upper extreme of normal limits.
- ☐ 3   **Mild** – Tends to give literal or personalised interpretations to the more difficult proverbs and may have some problems with concepts that are fairly abstract or remotely related.
- ☐ 4   **Moderate** – Often utilises a concrete mode. Has difficulty with most proverbs and some categories. Tends to be distracted by functional aspects and salient features.
- ☐ 5   **Moderate severe** – Deals primarily in a concrete mode, exhibiting difficulty with most proverbs and many categories.
- ☐ 6   **Severe** – Unable to grasp the abstract meaning of any proverbs or figurative expressions and can formulate classifications for only the most simple of similarities. Thinking is either vacuous or locked into functional aspects, salient features, and idiosyncratic interpretations.
- ☐ 7   **Extreme** – Can use only concrete modes of thinking. Shows no comprehension of proverbs, common metaphors or similes, and simple categories. Even salient and functional attributes do not serve as a basis for classification. This rating may apply to those who cannot interact even minimally with the examiner due to marked cognitive impairment.

14

N6. Lack of spontaneity and flow of conversation. Reduction in the normal flow of communication associated with apathy, avolition, defensiveness, or cognitive deficit. This is manifested by diminished fluidity and productivity of the verbal-interactional process. **Basis for rating:** cognitive-verbal processes observed during the course of interview.

- ☐ 1 **Absent** – Definition does not apply.
- ☐ 2 **Minimal** – Questionable pathology; may be at the upper extreme of normal limits.
- ☐ 3 **Mild** – Conversation shows little initiative. Patient's answers tend to be brief and unembellished, requiring direct and leading questions by the interviewer.
- ☐ 4 **Moderate** – Conversation lacks free flow and appears uneven or halting. Leading questions are frequently needed to elicit adequate responses and proceed with conversation.
- ☐ 5 **Moderate severe** – Patient shows a marked lack of spontaneity and openness, replying to the interviewer's questions with only one or two brief sentences.
- ☐ 6 **Severe** – Patient's responses are limited mainly to a few words or short phrases intended to avoid or curtail communication. (e.g. 'I don't know,' 'I'm not at liberty to say.') Conversation is seriously impaired as a result, and the interview is highly unproductive.
- ☐ 7 **Extreme** – Verbal output is restricted to, at most, an occasional utterance, making
- 15   conversation not possible.

N7. Stereotyped thinking. Decreased fluidity, spontaneity, and flexibility of thinking, as evidenced in rigid, repetitious, or barren thought content. **Basis for rating:** cognitive-verbal processes observed during the interview.

- ☐ 1 **Absent** – Definition does not apply.
- ☐ 2 **Minimal** – Questionable pathology; may be at the upper extreme of normal limits.
- ☐ 3 **Mild** – Some rigidity shown in attitudes or beliefs. Patient may refuse to consider alternative positions or have difficulty in shifting from one idea to another.
- ☐ 4 **Moderate** – Conversation revolves around a recurrent theme, resulting in difficulty in shifting to a new topic.
- ☐ 5 **Moderate severe** – Thinking is rigid and repetitious to the point that, despite the interviewer's efforts, conversation is limited to only two or three dominating topics.
- ☐ 6 **Severe** – Uncontrolled repetition of demands, statements, ideas, or questions which severely impairs conversation.
- ☐ 7 **Extreme** – Thinking, behaviour, and conversation are dominated by constant repetition of
- 16   fixed ideas or limited phrases, leading to gross rigidity, inappropriateness, and restrictiveness of patient's communication.

GENERAL PSYCHOPATHOLOGY SCALE (G)

G1. Somatic concern. Physical complaints or beliefs about bodily illness or malfunctions. This may range from a vague sense of ill-being to clear-cut delusions of catastrophic physical disease. **Basis for rating:** thought content expressed in the interview.

- ☐ 1 **Absent** – Definition does not apply.
- ☐ 2 **Minimal** – Questionable pathology; may be at the upper extreme of normal limits.
- ☐ 3 **Mild** – Distinctly concerned about health or somatic issues, as evidenced by occasional questions and desire for reassurance.
- ☐ 4 **Moderate** – Complains about poor health or bodily malfunction, but there is no delusional conviction, and overconcern can be allayed by reassurance.
- ☐ 5 **Moderate severe** – Patient expresses numerous or frequent complaints about physical illness or bodily malfunction, or else patient reveals one or two clear-cut delusions involving these themes but is not preoccupied by them.
- ☐ 6 **Severe** – Patient is preoccupied by one or a few clear-cut delusions about physical disease or organic malfunction, but affect is not fully immersed in these themes, and thoughts can be diverted by the interviewer with some effort.
- ☐ 7 **Extreme** – Numerous and frequently reported somatic delusions, or only a few somatic
- 17 delusions of a catastrophic nature, which totally dominate the patient's affect and thinking.

G2. Anxiety. Subjective experience of nervousness, worry, apprehension, or restlessness, ranging from excessive concern about the present or future to feelings of panic. **Basis for rating:** verbal report during the course of interview and corresponding physical manifestations.

- ☐ 1 **Absent** – Definition does not apply.
- ☐ 2 **Minimal** – Questionable pathology; may be at the upper extreme of normal limits.
- ☐ 3 **Mild** – Expresses some worry, overconcern, or subjective restlessness, but no somatic and behavioural consequences are reported or evidenced.
- ☐ 4 **Moderate** – Patient reports distinct symptoms of nervousness, which are reflected in mild physical manifestations such as fine hand tremor and excessive perspiration.
- ☐ 5 **Moderate severe** – Patient reports serious problems of anxiety which have significant physical and behavioural consequences, such as marked tension, poor concentration, palpitations, or impaired sleep.
- ☐ 6 **Severe** – Subjective state of almost constant fear associated with phobias, marked restlessness, or numerous somatic manifestations.
- ☐ 7 **Extreme** – Patient's life is seriously disrupted by anxiety, which is present almost constantly
- 18 and, at times, reaches panic proportion or is manifested in actual panic attacks.

G3. Guilt feelings. Sense of remorse or self-blame for real or imagined misdeeds in the past. **Basis for rating:** verbal report of guilt feelings during the course of interview and the influence on attitudes and thoughts.

- ☐ 1 **Absent** – Definition does not apply.
- ☐ 2 **Minimal** – Questionable pathology; may be at the upper extreme of normal limits.
- ☐ 3 **Mild** – Questioning elicits a vague sense of self-blame for a minor incident, but the patient clearly is not overly concerned.
- ☐ 4 **Moderate** – Patient expresses distinct concern over his responsibility for a real incident in his life but is not preoccupied with it, and attitude and behaviour are essentially unaffected.
- ☐ 5 **Moderate severe** – Patient expresses a strong sense of guilt associated with self-deprecation or the belief that he deserves punishment. The guilt feelings may have a delusional basis, may be volunteered spontaneously, may be a source of preoccupation and/or depressed mood, and cannot be allayed readily by the interviewer.
- ☐ 6 **Severe** – Strong ideas of guilt take on a delusional quality and lead to an attitude of hopelessness or worthlessness. The patient believes he should receive harsh sanctions for the misdeeds and may even regard his current life situation as such punishment.
- ☐ 7 **Extreme** – Patient's life is dominated by unshakeable delusions of guilt, for which he feels
- 19 deserving of drastic punishment, such as life imprisonment, torture, or death. There may be associated suicidal thoughts or attribution of others' problems to one's own past misdeeds.

G4. Tension. Overt physical manifestations of fear, anxiety, and agitation, such as stiffness, tremor, profuse sweating, and restlessness. **Basis for rating:** verbal report attesting to anxiety and, thereupon, the severity of physical manifestations observed during the interview.

- ☐ 1 **Absent** – Definition does not apply.
- ☐ 2 **Minimal** – Questionable pathology; may be at the upper extreme of normal limits.
- ☐ 3 **Mild** – Posture and movements indicate slight apprehensiveness, such as minor rigidity, occasional restlessness, shifting of position, or fine rapid hand tremor.
- ☐ 4 **Moderate** – A clearly nervous appearance emerges from various manifestations, such as fidgety behaviour, obvious hand tremor, excessive perspiration, or nervous mannerisms.
- ☐ 5 **Moderate severe** – Pronounced tension is evidenced by numerous manifestations, such as nervous shaking, profuse sweating, and restlessness, but conduct in the interview is not significantly affected.
- ☐ 6 **Severe** – Pronounced tension to the point that interpersonal interactions are disrupted. The patient, for example, may be constantly fidgeting, unable to sit still for long, or show hyperventilation.
- ☐ 7 **Extreme** – Marked tension is manifested by signs of panic or gross motor acceleration, such
- 20 as rapid restless pacing and inability to remain seated for longer than a minute, which makes sustained conversation not possible.

G5. Mannerisms and posturing. Unnatural movements or posture as characterised by an awkward, stilted, disorganised or bizarre appearance. **Basis for rating:** observation of physical manifestations during the course of interview as well as reports from primary care workers or family.

- ☐ 1 **Absent** – Definition does not apply.
- ☐ 2 **Minimal** – Questionable pathology; may be at the upper extreme of normal limits.
- ☐ 3 **Mild** – Slight awkwardness in movements or minor rigidity of posture.
- ☐ 4 **Moderate** – Movements are notably awkward or disjointed, or an unnatural posture is maintained for brief periods.
- ☐ 5 **Moderate severe** – Occasional bizarre rituals, or contorted posture are observed, or an abnormal position is sustained for extended periods.
- ☐ 6 **Severe** – Frequent repetition of bizarre rituals, mannerism, or stereotyped movements, or a contorted posture is sustained for extended periods.
- ☐ 7 **Extreme** – Functioning is seriously impaired by virtually constant involvement in ritualistic, 21 manneristic, or stereotyped movements or by an unnatural fixed posture which is sustained for most of the time.

G6. Depression. Feelings of sadness, discouragement, helplessness, and pessimism. **Basis for rating:** verbal report of depressed mood during the course of interview and its observed influence on attitude and behaviour.

- ☐ 1 **Absent** – Definition does not apply.
- ☐ 2 **Minimal** – Questionable pathology; may be at the upper extreme of normal limits.
- ☐ 3 **Mild** – Expresses some sadness or discouragement only on questioning, but there is no evidence of depression in general attitude or demeanour.
- ☐ 4 **Moderate** – Distinct feelings of sadness or hopelessness, which may be spontaneously divulged, but depressed mood has no major impact on behaviour or social functioning, and the patient usually can be cheered up.
- ☐ 5 **Moderate severe** – Distinctly depressed mood is associated with obvious sadness, pessimism, loss of social interest, psychomotor retardation, and some interference in appetite and sleep. The patient cannot be easily cheered up.
- ☐ 6 **Severe** – Markedly depressed mood is associated with sustained feelings of misery, occasional crying, hopelessness, and worthlessness. In addition, there is major interference in appetite and/or sleep as well as in normal motor and social functions, with possible signs of self-neglect.
- ☐ 7 **Extreme** – Depressive feelings seriously interfere in most major functions. The 22 manifestations include frequent crying, pronounced somatic symptoms, impaired concentration, psychomotor retardation, social disinterest, self-neglect, possible depressive or nihilistic delusions, and/or possible suicidal thoughts or action.

G7. Motor retardation. Reduction in motor activity as reflected in slowing or lessening of movements and speech, diminished responsiveness to stimuli, and reduced body tone. **Basis for rating:** manifestations during the course of interview as well as reports by primary care workers or family.

- ☐ 1 **Absent** – Definition does not apply.
- ☐ 2 **Minimal** – Questionable pathology; may be at the upper extreme of normal limits.
- ☐ 3 **Mild** – Slight but noticeable diminution in rate of movements and speech. Patient may be somewhat underproductive in conversation and gestures.
- ☐ 4 **Moderate** – Patient is clearly slow in movements, and speech may be characterised by poor productivity, including long response latency, extended pauses, or slow pace.
- ☐ 5 **Moderate severe** – A marked reduction in motor activity renders communication highly unproductive or delimits functioning in social and occupational situations. Patient can usually be found sitting or lying down.
- ☐ 6 **Severe** – Movements are extremely slow, resulting in a minimum of activity and speech. Essentially the day is spent sitting idly or lying down.
- ☐ 7 **Extreme** – Patient is almost completely immobile and virtually unresponsive to external
- 23   stimuli.

G8. Uncooperativeness. Active refusal to comply with the will of significant others, including the interviewer, hospital staff, or family, which may be associated with distrust, defensiveness, stubbornness, negativism, rejection of authority, hostility, or belligerence. **Basis for rating:** interpersonal behaviour observed during the course of interview as well as reports by primary care workers or family.

- ☐ 1 **Absent** – Definition does not apply.
- ☐ 2 **Minimal** – Questionable pathology; may be at the upper extreme of normal limits.
- ☐ 3 **Mild** – Complies with an attitude of resentment, impatience, or sarcasm. May inoffensively object to sensitive probing during the interview.
- ☐ 4 **Moderate** – Occasional outright refusal to comply with normal social demands, such as making own bed, attending scheduled programs, etc. The patient may project a hostile, defensive, or negative attitude but usually can be worked with.
- ☐ 5 **Moderate severe** – Patient frequently is incompliant with the demands of his milieu and may be characterised by others as an 'outcast' or having 'a serious attitude problem.' Uncooperativeness is reflected in obvious defensiveness or irritability with the interviewer and possible unwillingness to address many questions.
- ☐ 6 **Severe** – Patient is highly uncooperative, negativistic, and possibly also belligerent. Refuses to comply with most social demands and may be unwilling to initiate or conclude the full interview.
- ☐ 7 **Extreme** – Active resistance seriously impacts on virtually all major areas of functioning.
- 24   Patient may refuse to join in any social activities, tend to personal hygiene, converse with family or staff, and participate even briefly in an interview.

G9. Unusual thought content. Thinking characterised by strange, fantastic, or bizarre ideas, ranging from those which are remote or atypical to those which are distorted, illogical, and patiently absurd. **Basis for rating:** thought content expressed during the course of the interview.

☐ 1 **Absent** – Definition does not apply.
☐ 2 **Minimal** – Questionable pathology; may be at the upper extreme of normal limits.
☐ 3 **Mild** – Thought content is somewhat peculiar or idiosyncratic, or familiar ideas are framed in an odd context.
☐ 4 **Moderate** – Ideas are frequently distorted and occasionally seem quite bizarre.
☐ 5 **Moderate severe** – Patient expresses many strange and fantastic thoughts (e.g. being the adopted son of a king, being an escapee from death row) or some which are patently absurd (e.g. having hundreds of children, receiving messages from outer space through a tooth filling).
☐ 6 **Severe** – Patient expresses many illogical or absurd ideas or some which have a distinctly bizarre quality (e.g. having three heads, being a visitor from another planet).
☐ 7 **Extreme** – Thinking is replete with absurd, bizarre, and grotesque ideas.
25

G10. Disorientation. Lack of awareness of one's relationship to the milieu, including persons, place, and time, which may be due to confusion or withdrawal. **Basis for rating:** responses to interview questions on orientation.

☐ 1 **Absent** – Definition does not apply.
☐ 2 **Minimal** – Questionable pathology; may be at the upper extreme of normal limits.
☐ 3 **Mild** – General orientation is adequate but there is some difficulty with specifics. For example, patient knows his location but not the street address; knows hospital staff names but not their functions; knows the month but confuses the day of week with an adjacent day; or errs in the date by more than two days. There may be narrowing of interest evidenced by familiarity with the immediate but not extended milieu, such as ability to identify staff but not the Mayor, Governor, or President.
☐ 4 **Moderate** – Only partial success in recognising persons, places, and time. For example, patient knows he is in a hospital but not its name; knows the name of his city but not the borough or district; knows the name of his primary therapist but not many other direct care workers; knows the year and season but is not sure of the month.
☐ 5 **Moderate severe** – Considerable failure in recognising persons, places, and time. Patient has only a vague notion of where he is and seems unfamiliar with most people in his milieu. He may identify the year correctly or nearly so but not know the current month, day of week, or even the season.
☐ 6 **Severe** – Marked failure in recognising persons, place, and time. For example, patient has no knowledge of his whereabouts; confuses the date by more than one year; can name only one or two individuals in his current life.
☐ 7 **Extreme** – Patient appears completely disoriented with regard to persons, place, and time. There is gross confusion or total ignorance about one's location, the current year, and even the most familiar people, such as parents, spouse, friends, and primary therapist.
26

G11. Poor attention. Failure in focused alertness manifested by poor concentration, distractibility from internal and external stimuli, and difficulty in harnessing, sustaining, or shifting focus to new stimuli. **Basis for rating:** manifestations during the course of the interview.

☐ 1 **Absent** – Definition does not apply.
☐ 2 **Minimal** – Questionable pathology; may be at the upper extreme of normal limits.
☐ 3 **Mild** – Limited concentration evidenced by occasional vulnerability to distraction or faltering attention toward the end of the interview.
☐ 4 **Moderate** – Conversation is affected by the tendency to be easily distracted, difficulty in long sustaining concentration on a given topic, or problems in shifting attention to new topics.
☐ 5 **Moderate severe** – Conversation is seriously hampered by poor concentration, distractibility, and difficulty in shifting focus appropriately.
☐ 6 **Severe** – Patient's attention can be harnessed for only brief moments or with great effort, due to marked distraction by internal or external stimuli.
☐ 7 **Extreme** – Attention is so disrupted that even brief conversation is not possible.
27

G12. Lack of judgement and insight. Impaired awareness or understanding of one's own psychiatric condition and life situation. This is evidenced by failure to recognise past or present psychiatric illness or symptoms, denial of need for psychiatric hospitalisation or treatment, decisions characterised by poor anticipation of consequences, and unrealistic short-term and long-range planning. **Basis for rating:** thought content expressed during the interview.

☐ 1 **Absent** – Definition does not apply.
☐ 2 **Minimal** – Questionable pathology; may be at the upper extreme of normal limits.
☐ 3 **Mild** – Recognises having a psychiatric disorder but clearly underestimates its seriousness, the implications for treatment, or the importance of taking measures to avoid relapse. Future planning may be poorly conceived.
☐ 4 **Moderate** – Patient shows only a vague or shallow recognition of illness. There may be fluctuations in acknowledgement of being ill or little awareness of major symptoms which are present, such as delusions, disorganised thinking, suspiciousness, and social withdrawal. The patient may rationalise the need for treatment in terms of its relieving lesser symptoms, such as anxiety, tension, and sleep difficulty.
☐ 5 **Moderate severe** – Acknowledges past but not present psychiatric disorder. If challenged, the patient may concede the presence of some unrelated or insignificant symptoms, which tend to be explained away by gross misinterpretation or delusional thinking. The need for psychiatric treatment similarly goes unrecognised.
☐ 6 **Severe** – Patient denies ever having had a psychiatric disorder. He disavows the presence of any psychiatric symptoms in the past or present and, though compliant, denies the need for treatment and hospitalisation.
☐ 7 **Extreme** – Emphatic denial of past and present psychiatric illness. Current hospitalisation and treatment are given a delusional interpretation (e.g. as punishment for misdeeds, as persecution by tormentors, etc.), and the patient may thus refuse to cooperate with therapists, medication, or other aspects of treatment.
28

G13. Disturbance of volition. Disturbance in the wilful initiation, sustenance, and control of one's thoughts, behaviour, movements, and speech. **Basis for rating:** thought content and behaviour manifested in the course of the interview.

☐ 1   **Absent** – Definition does not apply.
☐ 2   **Minimal** – Questionable pathology; may be at the upper extreme of normal limits.
☐ 3   **Mild** – There is evidence of some indecisiveness in conversation and thinking, which may impede verbal and cognitive processes to a minor extent.
☐ 4   **Moderate** – Patient is often ambivalent and shows clear difficulty in reaching decisions. Conversation may be marred by alternation in thinking, and in consequence verbal and cognitive functioning are clearly impaired.
☐ 5   **Moderate severe** – Disturbance of volition interferes in thinking as well as behaviour. Patient shows pronounced indecision that impedes the initiation and continuation of social and motor activities, and which also may be evidenced in halting speech.
☐ 6   **Severe** – Disturbance of volition interferes in the execution of simple, automatic motor functions, such as dressing and grooming, and markedly affects speech.
☐ 7   **Extreme** – Almost complete failure of volition is manifested by gross inhibition of
29   movement and speech, resulting in immobility and/or mutism.

G14. Poor impulse control. Disordered regulation and control of action on inner urges, resulting in sudden, unmodulated, arbitrary, or misdirected discharge of tension and emotions without concern about consequences. **Basis for rating:** behaviour during the course of interview and reported by primary care workers or family.

☐ 1   **Absent** – Definition does not apply.
☐ 2   **Minimal** – Questionable pathology; may be at the upper extreme of normal limits.
☐ 3   **Mild** – Patient tends to be easily angered and frustrated when facing stress or denied gratification but rarely acts on impulse.
☐ 4   **Moderate** – Patient gets angered and verbally abusive with minimal provocation. May be occasionally threatening, destructive, or have one or two episodes involving physical confrontation or a minor brawl.
☐ 5   **Moderate severe** – Patient exhibits repeated impulsive episodes involving verbal abuse, destruction of property, or physical threats. There may be one or two episodes involving serious assault, for which the patient requires isolation, physical restraint, or p.r.n. sedation.
☐ 6   **Severe** – Patient frequently is impulsively aggressive, threatening, demanding, and destructive, without any apparent consideration of consequences. Shows assaultive behaviour and may also be sexually offensive and possibly respond behaviourally to hallucinatory commands.
☐ 7   **Extreme** – Patient exhibits homicidal attacks, sexual assaults, repeated brutality, or self-
30   destructive behaviour. Requires constant direct supervision or external constraints because of inability to control dangerous impulses.

G15. Preoccupation. Absorption with internally generated thoughts and feelings and with autistic experiences to the detriment of reality orientation and adaptive behaviour. **Basis for rating:** interpersonal behaviour observed during the course of the interview.

☐ 1   **Absent** – Definition does not apply.

☐ 2   **Minimal** – Questionable pathology; may be at the upper extreme of normal limits.

☐ 3   **Mild** – Excessive involvement with personal needs or problems, such that conversation veers back to egocentric themes and there is diminished concern exhibited toward others.

☐ 4   **Moderate** – Patient occasionally appears self-absorbed, as if daydreaming or involved with internal experiences, which interferes with communication to a minor extent.

☐ 5   **Moderate severe** – Patient often appears to be engaged in autistic experiences, as evidenced by behaviours that significantly intrude on social and communicational functions, such as the presence of a vacant stare, muttering or talking to oneself, or involvement with stereotyped motor patterns.

☐ 6   **Severe** – Marked preoccupation with autistic experiences, which seriously delimits concentration, ability to converse, and orientation to the milieu. The patient frequently may be observed smiling, laughing, muttering, talking, or shouting to himself.

☐ 7   **Extreme** – Gross absorption with autistic experiences, which profoundly affects all major
31   realms of behaviour. The patient constantly may be responding verbally and behaviourally to hallucinations and show little awareness of other people or the external milieu.

G16. Active social avoidance. Diminished social involvement associated with unwarranted fear, hostility, or distrust. **Basis for rating:** reports of social functioning by primary care workers or family.

☐ 1   **Absent** – Definition does not apply.

☐ 2   **Minimal** – Questionable pathology; may be at the upper extreme of normal limits.

☐ 3   **Mild** – Patient seems ill at ease in the presence of others and prefers to spend time alone, although he participates in social functions when required.

☐ 4   **Moderate** – Patient begrudgingly attends all or most social activities but may need to be persuaded or may terminate prematurely on account of anxiety, suspiciousness, or hostility.

☐ 5   **Moderate severe** – Patient fearfully or angrily keeps away from many social interactions despite others' efforts to engage him. Tends to spend unstructured time alone.

☐ 6   **Severe** – Patient participates in very few social activities because of fear, hostility, or distrust. When approached, the patient shows a strong tendency to break off interactions, and generally he appears to isolate himself from others.

☐ 7   **Extreme** – Patient cannot be engaged in social activities because of pronounced fears,
32   hostility, or persecutory delusions. To the extent possible, he avoids all interactions and remains isolated from others.

Patients must score 120 on the total of all items of the PANSS to be included in the trial

TOTAL SCORE   33   ☐☐

Reproduced from Kay et al (1987) *Schizophrenia Bull* **13**, 261–76.

BPRS

Please enter the score for the term which best describes the subject's condition

1. SOMATIC CONCERN
- ☐ 0 Not present
- ☐ 1 Very mild
- ☐ 2 Mild
- ☐ 3 Moderate
- ☐ 4 Moderately severe
- ☐ 5 Severe
- ☐ 6 Extremely severe

3

2. ANXIETY
- ☐ 0 Not present
- ☐ 1 Very mild
- ☐ 2 Mild
- ☐ 3 Moderate
- ☐ 4 Moderately severe
- ☐ 5 Severe
- ☐ 6 Extremely severe

4

3. EMOTIONAL WITHDRAWAL
- ☐ 0 Not present
- ☐ 1 Very mild
- ☐ 2 Mild
- ☐ 3 Moderate
- ☐ 4 Moderately severe
- ☐ 5 Severe
- ☐ 6 Extremely severe

5

4. CONCEPTUAL DISORGANISATION
- ☐ 0 Not present
- ☐ 1 Very mild
- ☐ 2 Mild
- ☐ 3 Moderate
- ☐ 4 Moderately severe
- ☐ 5 Severe
- ☐ 6 Extremely severe

6

5. GUILT FEELINGS
- ☐ 0 Not present
- ☐ 1 Very mild
- ☐ 2 Mild
- ☐ 3 Moderate
- ☐ 4 Moderately severe
- ☐ 5 Severe
- ☐ 6 Extremely severe

7

6. TENSION
- ☐ 0 Not present
- ☐ 1 Very mild
- ☐ 2 Mild
- ☐ 3 Moderate
- ☐ 4 Moderately severe
- ☐ 5 Severe
- ☐ 6 Extremely severe

8

7. MANNERISMS AND POSTURING
- ☐ 0 Not present
- ☐ 1 Very mild
- ☐ 2 Mild
- ☐ 3 Moderate
- ☐ 4 Moderately severe
- ☐ 5 Severe
- ☐ 6 Extremely severe

9

8. GRANDIOSITY
- ☐ 0 Not present
- ☐ 1 Very mild
- ☐ 2 Mild
- ☐ 3 Moderate
- ☐ 4 Moderately severe
- ☐ 5 Severe
- ☐ 6 Extremely severe

10

9. DEPRESSIVE MOOD
- ☐ 0   Not present
- ☐ 1   Very mild
- ☐ 2   Mild
- ☐ 3   Moderate
- ☐ 4   Moderately severe
- ☐ 5   Severe
- ☐ 6   Extremely severe

11

10. HOSTILITY
- ☐ 0   Not present
- ☐ 1   Very mild
- ☐ 2   Mild
- ☐ 3   Moderate
- ☐ 4   Moderately severe
- ☐ 5   Severe
- ☐ 6   Extremely severe

12

11. SUSPICIOUSNESS
- ☐ 0   Not present
- ☐ 1   Very mild
- ☐ 2   Mild
- ☐ 3   Moderate
- ☐ 4   Moderately severe
- ☐ 5   Severe
- ☐ 6   Extremely severe

13

12. HALLUCINATORY BEHAVIOUR
- ☐ 0   Not present
- ☐ 1   Very mild
- ☐ 2   Mild
- ☐ 3   Moderate
- ☐ 4   Moderately severe
- ☐ 5   Severe
- ☐ 6   Extremely severe

14

13. MOTOR RETARDATION
- ☐ 0   Not present
- ☐ 1   Very mild
- ☐ 2   Mild
- ☐ 3   Moderate
- ☐ 4   Moderately severe
- ☐ 5   Severe
- ☐ 6   Extremely severe

15

14. UNCOOPERATIVENESS
- ☐ 0   Not present
- ☐ 1   Very mild
- ☐ 2   Mild
- ☐ 3   Moderate
- ☐ 4   Moderately severe
- ☐ 5   Severe
- ☐ 6   Extremely severe

16

15. UNUSUAL THOUGHT CONTENT
- ☐ 0   Not present
- ☐ 1   Very mild
- ☐ 2   Mild
- ☐ 3   Moderate
- ☐ 4   Moderately severe
- ☐ 5   Severe
- ☐ 6   Extremely severe

17

16. BLUNTED AFFECT
- ☐ 0   Not present
- ☐ 1   Very mild
- ☐ 2   Mild
- ☐ 3   Moderate
- ☐ 4   Moderately severe
- ☐ 5   Severe
- ☐ 6   Extremely severe

18

17. EXCITEMENT
- ☐ 0   Not present
- ☐ 1   Very mild
- ☐ 2   Mild
- ☐ 3   Moderate
- ☐ 4   Moderately severe
- ☐ 5   Severe
- ☐ 6   Extremely severe

19

18. DISORIENTATION
- ☐ 0   Not present
- ☐ 1   Very mild
- ☐ 2   Mild
- ☐ 3   Moderate
- ☐ 4   Moderately severe
- ☐ 5   Severe
- ☐ 6   Extremely severe

20

TOTAL SCORE ☐ ☐ ☐

Reproduced from Overall and Graham (1962) *Psychological Reports* **10**, 799–812.

Clinical Global Impression Scale (CGI)

1. Considering your total experience with similar patients, how mentally ill is the patient at this time?
   1 Normal, not at all ill
   2 Borderline
   3 Mildly ill
   4 Moderately ill
   5 Markedly ill
   6 Severely ill
   7 Among the most extremely ill

2. Compared to his/her condition since recruitment, how much has changed?
   1 Very much improved
   2 Much improved
   3 Minimally improved
   4 No change
   5 Minimally worse
   6 Much worse
   7 Very much worse
   8 Not applicable

3. Select the term that best characterises the therapeutic effect of this particular treatment
   1 Marked–vast improvement. Complete or nearly complete remission of all symptoms.
   2 Moderate/decided improvement
   3 Minimal–slight improvement. Partial remission of symptoms
   4 Unchanged
   5 Worse–increase in symptoms
   6 Not applicable

Reproduced from Guy (1976) Assessment Manual for Psychopharmacology Revised. US Dept Health Education and Welfare, pp. 218–22.

Global Assessment Scale (GAS)

Subject's lowest level of functioning in the last week by selecting the lowest range which describes his functioning on a high–low continuum of mental health-illness. For example, a subject whose behaviour is 'considerably influenced by delusions' should be given a rating in that range (21–30) even though he has 'major impediment in several areas' (range 31–40). Use intermediary as appropriate (e.g. 35, 58, 63). Rate actual functioning independent of whether or not subject is receiving help and/or medication and may be helped by this or some other form of treatment.

100–91	No symptoms, superior functioning in a wide range of activities, life's problems never seem to get out of hand, is sought out by others because of his warmth and integrity.
90–81	Transient symptoms may occur, but good functioning in all areas, interested and involved in a wide range of activities, socially effective, generally satisfied with life, 'everyday' worries never seem to get out of hand.
80–71	Minimal symptoms may be present, but no more than slight impairment in functioning, varying degrees of 'everyday' worries and problems that sometimes get out of hand.
70–61	Some mild symptoms (e.g. depressive mood and mild insomnia) OR some difficulty in several areas of functioning, but generally functioning pretty well, has some meaningful interpersonal relationships and most untrained people would not consider him 'sick'.
60–51	Moderate symptoms OR generally functioning with some difficulty (e.g. few friends and flat affect, depressed mood and pathological self-doubt, euphoric mood and pressure of speech, moderately severe antisocial behaviour).
50–41	Any serious symptomatology or impairment in functioning that most clinicians would think obviously requires treatment or attention (e.g. suicidal preoccupation or gesture, severe obsessional rituals, frequent anxiety attacks, serious antisocial behaviour, compulsive drinking).
40–31	Major impairment in several areas, such as work, family relations, judgement, thinking, or mood (e.g. depressed woman avoids friends, neglects family, unable to do housework) OR some impairment in reality testing or communication (e.g. speech is at times obscure, illogical, or irrelevant) OR single serious suicide attempt.
30–21	Unable to function in almost all areas (e.g. stays in bed all day) OR behaviour is considerably influenced by delusions or hallucinations, OR serious impairment in communication (e.g. sometimes incoherent or unresponsive) or judgement (e.g. acts grossly inappropriately).
20–11	Needs some supervision to prevent hurting self or others, or to maintain minimal personal hygiene (e.g. repeated suicide attempts, frequently violent, manic excitement, smears faeces), OR gross impairment in communications (e.g. largely incoherent or mute).
10–1	Needs constant supervision for several days to prevent hurting self or others, or makes no attempt to maintain minimal personal hygiene.

Reproduced by permission of the American Medical Association from Endicott et al (1976) *Arch Gen Psychiatry* **33**, 766–71.

Health of the Nation Outcome Scales (HONOS)

1. Overactive, aggressive, disruptive or agitated **behaviour**
   - Include such behaviour due to any cause, e.g. drugs, alcohol, dementia, psychosis, depression, etc.
   - Do not include bizarre behaviour rated on scale 6
   - 0 No problem.
   - 1 Irritability, quarrels, restlessness, etc. not requiring action.
   - 2 Includes aggressive gestures, pushing or pestering others; threats or verbal aggression; lesser damage to property (e.g. broken cups, windows); marked overactivity or agitation.
   - 3 Physical aggressive to others or animals (short of rating 4); threatening manner; more serious over activity or destruction of property.
   - 4 At least one serious attack on others or on animals; destructive of property (e.g. fire setting); serious intimidation or obscene behaviour.
   - 9 Unknown.

     □

2. Non-accidental self-injury
   - Do not include accidental self-injury due to dementia or severe learning disability; the cognitive problem is rated at scale 4 and the injury at scale 5.
   - Do not include illness or injury as a direct consequence of alcohol or drug use rated at scale 3 (e.g. cirrhosis of liver or injury resulting from drink driving are related at scale 5).
   - 0 No problems.
   - 1 Fleeting thought about ending it all but little risk during the period related; no self-harm.
   - 2 Mild risk during the period rated; includes non-hazardous self-harm (e.g. wrist scratching).
   - 3 Moderate to serious risk of deliberate self-harm during the period rated; includes preparatory acts (e.g. collecting tablets).
   - 4 Serious suicidal attempts and/or serious deliberate self-injury during the rated period.
   - 9 Unknown.

     □

3. Problem drinking or drug taking
   - Do not include aggressive/destructive behaviour due to alcohol or drug use, rated at scale 1.
   - Do not include physical illness or disability due to alcohol or drug use, rated at scale 5.
   - 0 No problems.
   - 1 Some overindulgence but within social norms.
   - 2 Loss of control of drinking or drug taking, but not seriously addicted.
   - 3 Marked craving or dependence on alcohol or drugs with frequent loss of control; risk taking behaviour under the influence.
   - 4 Incapacitated by alcohol/drug problem.
   - 9 Unknown.

     □

4. Cognitive problems
   - Include problems of memory, orientation and understanding associated with any disorder: learning disability, dementia, schizophrenia, etc.
   - Do not include temporary problems (e.g. hangover) resulting from drug or alcohol misuse.
   - 0 No problems.
   - 1 Minor problems, with memory or understanding (e.g. forgets names occasionally).
   - 2 Mild but definite problem (e.g. has lost the way in a familiar place or failed to recognise a familiar person); sometimes mixed up about simple decisions.

    3   Marked disorientation in time, place or person; bewildered by everyday events; speech is sometimes incoherent; mental slowing.

    4   Severe disorientation (e.g. unable to recognise relatives); at risk of accidents; speech incomprehensible; clouding or stupor.

    9   Unknown.

                   ☐

                   ☐

5.   Physical illness or disability problems
- Include illness or disability from any cause that limits or prevents movement, or impairs sight, or hearing or otherwise interferes with personal functioning.
- Include side-effects of medication; effects of drug/alcohol; physical disabilities resulting from accidents or self-harm associated with cognitive problems, drink–driving, etc.

    0   No problems.

    1   Minor health problems, e.g. cold, non serious fall.

    2   Physical health problems impose mild restriction on mobility and activity.

    3   Moderate degree of restriction on activity due to physical health problems.

    4   Severe or complete incapacity due to physical health problems.

    9   Unknown.

                   ☐

6.   Problems associated with hallucinations and delusions
- Include hallucinations and delusions irrespective of diagnosis.
- Include odd or bizarre behaviour associated with hallucinations or delusions.
- Do not include aggressive or destructive behaviour attributed to hallucinations or delusions attributed to scale 1.

    0   No evidence of hallucinations or delusions.

    1   Somewhat odd or eccentric beliefs not in keeping with cultural norms.

    2   Delusions or hallucinations (e.g. voice, visions) are present but there is little distress to patient or manifestation in bizarre behaviour, i.e. clinically present but mild.

    3   Marked preoccupation with delusions or hallucinations causing much distress and/or manifested in obviously bizarre behaviour, i.e. moderately severe problem.

    4   Mental state and behaviour are seriously and adversely affected by delusions or hallucinations with severe impact on patient.

    9   Unknown.

                   ☐

7.   Problems associated with depressed mood
- Do not include overactivity or agitation, rated at scale 1.
- Do not include suicidal ideation (scale 2).
- Do not include delusions or hallucinations (scale 6).

    0   No problem of depressed mood.

    1   Gloomy; minor changes in mood.

    2   Mild but definite depression and distress (e.g. feelings of guilt; loss of self-esteem).

    3   Depression with inappropriate self-blame; preoccupied with feelings of guilt.

    4   Severe or very severe depression with guilt and self-accusation.

    9   Unknown.

                   ☐

8.   Other mental and behavioural problems
- Rate only the most severe clinical problem not considered in items 6 and 7 as follows.
- Specify the type of problem by entering the appropriate letter.

- A phobic; B anxiety; C OCD; D mental strain/tension; E dissociative; F somatoform; G eating; H sleep; I sexual; J other, specify.
  - 0 No problem.
  - 1 Minor problem only.
  - 2 A problem is clinically present at a mild level (e.g. the patient has a degree of control).
  - 3 Occasional severe attack of distress, with loss of control (e.g. has to avoid anxiety-provoking situations altogether, call a neighbour for help, etc.) i.e. moderately severe level of problem.
  - 4 Severe problem dominates most activities.
  - 9 Unknown.

☐

9. Problems with relationships
- Rate the patient's most severe problem associated with active or passive withdrawal from social relationships, and/or non-supportive, destructive or self-damaging relationships.
  - 0 No problem.
  - 1 Minor non-clinical problem.
  - 2 Definite problem in making or sustaining supportive relationships: patient complains and/or problems are evident to others.
  - 3 Persisting major problems due to active or passive withdrawal from social relationships and/or to relationships that provide little or no comfort or support.
  - 4 Severe and distressing social isolation due to inability to communicate socially and/or withdrawal from social relationships.
  - 9 Unknown.

☐

10. Problems with activities of daily living
- Rate the overall level of functioning in activities of daily living, e.g. problems eating, washing, dressing, toilet, budgeting, organising where to live, occupation and recreation, mobility and use of transport, shopping, self-development.
- Include any lack of motivation for using self-help opportunities, since this contributes to a lower level of functioning.
  - 0 No problem in the period rated.
  - 1 Minor problem only, e.g. untidy, disorganised.
  - 2 Self-care adequate, but major lack of performance of one or more complex skills.
  - 3 Major problem in one or more areas of self-care (eating, washing, dressing, toilet) as well as major inability to perform several complex skills.
  - 4 Severe disability or incapacity in all or nearly all areas of self-care and complex skills.
  - 9 Unknown.

☐

11. Problems with living conditions
- Rate the overall severity of problems with the quality of basic living conditions and daily domestic routine.
- Are the basic necessities met (heat, light, hygiene)? If so, is there help to cope with disabilities and a choice of opportunity to use skills and develop new ones?
- Do not rate functional disability itself, rated in 10.
  - 0 Accommodation and living conditions acceptable; helpful in keeping any disability rated at scale 10 to the lowest possible level and supportive of self-help.
  - 1 Accommodation is reasonably acceptable although there are minor or transient problems (e.g. not ideal location, not preferred option, doesn't like food).
  - 2 Significant problems with one or more aspects of the accommodation and/or regime

(e.g. restricted choice, staff or household have little understanding of how to limit disability or how to help use or develop new or intact skills).

3   Distressing multiple problems with accommodation (e.g. some basic necessities absent); housing environment has minimal or no facilities to improve patient's independence.

4   Accommodation is unacceptable (e.g. lack of basic necessities, patient is at risk of eviction or roofless, or intolerable living conditions) making patients' problem worse.

9   Unknown.

☐

12. Problems with occupation and activities
* Rate the overall level of problem with quality of daytime environment. Is there help to cope with disabilities and opportunities for maintaining or improving occupational and recreational skills and activities? Consider factors such as stigma, lack of qualified staff, access to supportive facilities (e.g. staffing and equipment of day centres, workshops, social clubs, etc.).
* Rate patient's usual situation.

0   Patient's daytime environment is acceptable: helpful in keeping any disability rated at scale 10 to the lowest level possible.

1   Minor or temporary problems (e.g. late giros), reasonable facilities available but not always at desired times, etc.

2   Limited choice of activities; lack of reasonable tolerance (e.g. unfairly refused entry to public library or baths); handicapped by lack of permanent address; insufficient carer or professional support; helpful day setting available but for very limited hours.

3   Marked deficiency in skilled services available to help minimise level of existing disability; no opportunities to use intact or add new ones; unskilled care difficult to access.

4   Lack of any opportunity for daytime activities makes patient's problems worse.

9   Unknown.

☐
☐

Reproduced by permission of the Royal College of Psychiatrists from Wing et al (1998) *Br J Psychiatry* 172, 11–18.

The Calgary Depression Scale for Schizophrenia

Interviewer: Ask the first questions as written. Use follow-up probes or qualifiers at your discretion. Time frame refers to last 2 weeks unless stipulated.

NB: The last item, no. 9, is based on observations of the entire interview.

1. Depression: How would you describe your mood over the last 2 weeks? Do you keep reasonably cheerful or have you been very depressed or low spirited recently? In the last 2 weeks, how often have you (own words) every day? All day?

0. Absent

1. Mild	Expresses some sadness or discouragement on questioning
2. Moderate	Distinct depressed mood persisting up to half the time over last 2 weeks: present daily
3. Severe	Markedly depressed mood persisting daily over half the time, interfering with normal motor and social functioning.

3. Self-depreciation: What is your opinion of yourself compared to other people? Do you feel better, not as good or about the same as others? Do you feel inferior or even worthless?

0. Absent

1. Mild	Some inferiority; not amounting to feeling of worthlessness.
2. Moderate	Subject feels worthless, but less than 50% of the time.
3. Severe	Subject feels worthless more than 50% of the time. May be challenged to acknowledge otherwise.

2. Hopelessness: How do you see the future for yourself? Can you see any future? Or has life seemed quite hopeless? Have you given up or does there still seem some reason for trying?

0. Absent

1. Mild	Has at times felt hopeless over the last 2 weeks, but still has some degree of hope for the future.
2. Moderate	Persistent, moderate sense of hopelessness over last 2 weeks. Can be persuaded to acknowledge possibility of things being better.
3. Severe	Persisting and distressing sense of hopelessness.

4. Guilty ideas of reference: Do you have the feeling that you are being blamed for something or even wrongly accused? What about? (Do not include justifiable blame or accusations. Exclude delusions of guilt.)

0. Absent

1. Mild	Subject feels blamed but not accused less than 50% of the time.
2. Moderate	Persisting sense of being blamed, and/or occasional sense of being accused.
3. Severe	Persistent sense of being accused. When challenged, acknowledges that it is not so.

85

5. Pathological guilt: Do you tend to blame yourself for little things you may have done in the past? Do you think that you deserve to be so concerned about this?

0. Absent

1. Mild   Subject sometimes feels over guilty about some minor peccadillo, but less than 50% of the time.

2. Moderate   Subject usually (over 50% of the time) feels guilty about past actions, the significance of which he exaggerates.

3. Severe   Subject usually feels s/he is to blame for everything that has gone wrong, even when not his/her fault.

7. Early wakening: Do you wake earlier in the morning than is normal for you? How many times a week does this happen?

0. Absent   No early wakening.

1. Mild   Occasionally wakes (up to twice weekly) 1 hour or more before normal time to wake or alarm time.

2. Moderate   Often wakes early (up to 5 times weekly) 1 hour or more before normal time to wake or alarm.

3. Severe   Daily wakes 1 hour or more before normal time.

6. Morning depression: When you have felt depressed over the last 2 weeks have you noticed the depression being worse at any particular time of day?

0. Absent   No depression.

1. Mild   Depression present but no diurnal variation.

2. Moderate   Depression spontaneously mentioned to be worse in morning.

3. Severe   Depression markedly worse in a.m., with impaired functioning, which improves in p.m.

8. Suicide: Have you felt that life wasn't worth living? Did you ever feel like ending it all? What did you think you might do? Did you actually try?

0. Absent

1. Mild   Frequent thoughts of being better off dead, or occasional thoughts of suicide.

2. Moderate   Deliberately considered suicide with a plan, but made no attempt.

3. Severe   Suicidal attempt apparently designed to end in death (i.e. accidental discovery or inefficient means).

9. Observed depression: Based on interviewer's observations during the entire interview? The question 'Do you feel like crying?' used at aappropriate points in the interview, may elicit information useful to this observation.

0. Absent

1. Mild   Subject appears sad and mournful even during parts of the interview involving effectively neutral discussion.

2. Moderate   Subject appears sad and mournful throughout the interview, with gloomy monotonous voice and is tearful or close to tears at times.

3. Severe   Subject chokes on distressing topics, frequently sighs deeply and cries openly, or is persistently in a state of frozen misery if examiner is sure that this is present.

Reproduced by permission of the Royal College of Psychiatrists from Addington et al (1993) *Br J Psychiatry* 22, 39–44.

The Schizophrenia Quality of Life Scale (SQLS)

Your Quality of Life

We are interested in finding out about the quality of your life **OVER THE PAST SEVEN DAYS.** Please respond to all the following statements by ticking one box for each statement. Your responses will remain confidential.

1. I lack the energy to do things.
   Never ☐ Rarely ☐ Sometimes ☐ Often ☐ Always ☐

2. I am bothered by my shaking/trembling.
   Never ☐ Rarely ☐ Sometimes ☐ Often ☐ Always ☐

3. I feel unsteady walking.
   Never ☐ Rarely ☐ Sometimes ☐ Often ☐ Always ☐

4. I feel angry.
   Never ☐ Rarely ☐ Sometimes ☐ Often ☐ Always ☐

5. I am troubled by a dry mouth.
   Never ☐ Rarely ☐ Sometimes ☐ Often ☐ Always ☐

6. I can't be bothered to do things.
   Never ☐ Rarely ☐ Sometimes ☐ Often ☐ Always ☐

7. I worry about my future.
   Never ☐ Rarely ☐ Sometimes ☐ Often ☐ Always ☐

8. I feel lonely.
   Never ☐ Rarely ☐ Sometimes ☐ Often ☐ Always ☐

9. I feel hopeless.
   Never ☐ Rarely ☐ Sometimes ☐ Often ☐ Always ☐

10. My muscles get stiff.
    Never ☐ Rarely ☐ Sometimes ☐ Often ☐ Always ☐

11. I feel very jumpy and edgy.
    Never ☐ Rarely ☐ Sometimes ☐ Often ☐ Always ☐

12. I am able to carry out my day to day activities.
    Never ☐ Rarely ☐ Sometimes ☐ Often ☐ Always ☐

13. I take part in enjoyable activities.
    Never ☐ Rarely ☐ Sometimes ☐ Often ☐ Always ☐

14. I take things people say the wrong way.
    Never ☐ Rarely ☐ Sometimes ☐ Often ☐ Always ☐

15. I like to plan ahead.
    Never ☐ Rarely ☐ Sometimes ☐ Often ☐ Always ☐

16. I find it hard to concentrate.
    Never ☐ Rarely ☐ Sometimes ☐ Often ☐ Always ☐

17.	I tend to stay at home.	Never ☐	Rarely ☐	Sometimes ☐	Often ☐	Always ☐
18.	I find it difficult to mix with people.	Never ☐	Rarely ☐	Sometimes ☐	Often ☐	Always ☐
19.	I feel down and depressed.	Never ☐	Rarely ☐	Sometimes ☐	Often ☐	Always ☐
20.	I feel that I can cope.	Never ☐	Rarely ☐	Sometimes ☐	Often ☐	Always ☐
21.	My vision is blurred.	Never ☐	Rarely ☐	Sometimes ☐	Often ☐	Always ☐
22.	I feel very mixed up and unsure of myself.	Never ☐	Rarely ☐	Sometimes ☐	Often ☐	Always ☐
23.	My sleep is disturbed.	Never ☐	Rarely ☐	Sometimes ☐	Often ☐	Always ☐
24.	My feelings go up and down.	Never ☐	Rarely ☐	Sometimes ☐	Often ☐	Always ☐
25.	I get muscle twitches.	Never ☐	Rarely ☐	Sometimes ☐	Often ☐	Always ☐
26.	I am concerned that I won't get better.	Never ☐	Rarely ☐	Sometimes ☐	Often ☐	Always ☐
27.	I worry about things.	Never ☐	Rarely ☐	Sometimes ☐	Often ☐	Always ☐
28.	I feel that people tend to avoid me.	Never ☐	Rarely ☐	Sometimes ☐	Often ☐	Always ☐
29.	I get upset thinking about the past.	Never ☐	Rarely ☐	Sometimes ☐	Often ☐	Always ☐
30.	I get dizzy spells.	Never ☐	Rarely ☐	Sometimes ☐	Often ☐	Always ☐

Reproduced by permission of the Royal College of Psychiatrists from Wilkinson et al (2000) *Br J Psychiatry* 177, 42–6.

Simpson–Angus Scale (SAS)

Enter appropriate code in boxes below.

1. GAIT

SCORE

☐

0 = Normal
1 = Mild diminution in swing while the patient is walking
2 = Obvious diminution in swing suggesting shoulder rigidity
3 = Stiff gait with little or no arm swing noticeable
4 = Rigid gait with arms slightly pronated; or stooped–shuffling gait with propulsion and retropulsion
9 = Not rateable

2. ARM DROPPING

SCORE

☐

0 = Normal, free fall with loud slap and rebound
1 = Fall slowed slightly with less audible contact and little rebound
2 = Fall slowed, no rebound
3 = Marked slowing, no slap at all
4 = Arms fall as though against resistance: as though through glue
9 = Not rateable

3. SHOULDER SHAKING

SCORE

☐

0 = Normal
1 = Slight stiffness and resistance
2 = Moderate stiffness and resistance
3 = Marked rigidity with difficulty in passive movement
4 = Extreme stiffness and rigidity with almost a frozen joint
9 = Not rateable

4. ELBOW RIGIDITY

SCORE

☐

0 = Normal
1 = Slight stiffness and resistance
2 = Moderate stiffness and resistance
3 = Marked rigidity with difficulty in passive movement
4 = Extreme stiffness and rigidity with almost a frozen joint
9 = Not rateable

5. WRIST RIGIDITY

SCORE

☐

0 = Normal
1 = Slight stiffness and resistance
2 = Moderate stiffness and resistance
3 = Marked rigidity with difficulty in passive movement
4 = Extreme stiffness and rigidity with almost a frozen joint
9 = Not rateable

6. LEG PENDULOUSNESS

SCORE

☐

0 = The legs swing freely
1 = Slight diminution in the swing of the legs
2 = Moderate resistance to swing
3 = Marked resistance and damping of swing
4 = Complete absence of swing
9 = Not rateable

7. HEAD DROPPING

SCORE   **0** = The head falls completely with a good thump as it hits the table

☐   **1** = Slight slowing in fall, mainly noted by lack of slap as head meets the table
     2 = Moderate slowing in the fall quite noticeable to the eye
     3 = Head falls stiffly and slowly
     4 = Head does not reach examining table
     9 = Not rateable

8. GLABELLAR TAP

SCORE   **0** = 0–5 blinks

☐   **1** = 6–10 blinks
     2 = 11–15 blinks
     3 = 16–20 blinks
     4 = 21 or more blinks
     9 = Not rateable

9. TREMOR

SCORE   **0** = Normal

☐   **1** = Mild finger tremor, obvious to sight and touch
     2 = Tremor of hand or arm occurring spasmodically
     3 = Persistent tremor of one or more limbs
     4 = Whole body tremor
     9 = Not rateable

10. SALIVATION

SCORE   **0** = Normal

☐   **1** = Excess salivation so that pooling takes place if mouth is open and tongue is raised
     2 = Excess salivation is present and might occasionally result in difficulty speaking
     3 = Speaking with difficulty because of excess salivation
     4 = Frank drooling
     9 = Not rateable

Reproduced by permission of Blackwell Publishing from Simpson and Angus (1970) *Acta Psychiatr Scand* **212** (suppl.), 11–19.

Barnes Akathisia Rating Scale (BAS)

INSTRUCTIONS

Patient should be observed while seated, and then standing while engaged in neutral conversation (for a minimum of 2 minutes in each position). Symptoms observed in other situations, for example, while engaged in activity on the ward, may also be rated. Subsequently, the **subjective** phenomena should be elicited by direct questioning.

Put appropriate code in box below.

OBJECTIVE

0 = Normal, occasional fidgety movements of the limbs

1 = Presence of characteristic restless movements: shuffling or tramping movements of the legs and feet or swinging of one leg, while sitting, *and/or* rocking from foot to foot or 'walking on the spot' when standing, *but* movements present for less than half the time observed

2 = Observed phenomena, as described in (1) above, which are present for at least half the observation period

3 = Patient is constantly engaged in characteristic restless movements, *and/or* has the inability to remain seated or standing without walking or pacing, during the time observed

SUBJECTIVE

AWARENESS OF RESTLESSNESS

0 = Absence of inner restlessness

1 = Nonspecific sense of inner restlessness

2 = Patient is aware of an inability to keep the legs still, or a desire to move the legs, *and/or* complains of inner restlessness aggravated specifically by being required to stand still

3 = Awareness of an intense compulsion to move most of the time *and/or* reports a strong desire to walk or pace most of the time

DISTRESS RELATED TO RESTLESSNESS

0 = No distress

1 = Mild

2 = Moderate

3 = Severe

GLOBAL CLINICAL ASSESSMENT OF AKATHISIA

0 = *Absent* – no evidence of awareness of restlessness. Observation of characteristic movements of akathisia in the absence of a subjective report of inner restlessness or compulsive desire to move the legs should be classified as pseudoakathisia

1 = *Questionable* – nonspecific inner tension and fidgety movements

2 = *Mild akathisia* – awareness of restlessness in the legs *and/or* inner restlessness worse when required to stand still. Fidgety movements present, but characteristic restless movements of akathisia not necessarily observed. Condition causes little or no distress

3 = *Moderate akathisia* – awareness of restlessness as described for mild akathisia above, combined with characteristic restless movements such as rocking from foot to foot when standing. Patient finds the condition distressing

4 = *Marked akathisia* – subjective experience of restlessness includes a compulsive desire to walk or pace. However, the patient is able to remain seated for at least 5 minutes. The condition is obviously distressing

5 = *Severe akathisia* – the patient reports a strong compulsion to pace up and down most of the time. Unable to sit or lie down for more than a few minutes. Constant restlessness which is associated with intense distress and insomnia

Reproduced by permission of the Royal College of Psychiatrists from Barnes (1989) *Br J Psychiatry* **154**, 672–6.

Abnormal Involuntary Movement Scale (AIMS)

Instructions: Complete examination procedure before making ratings. When rating movements, rate highest severity observed and rate movements that occur upon activation one less than those observed spontaneously.
(Put appropriate code in boxes below)

FACIAL AND ORAL MOVEMENTS
1. **Muscles of facial expression**
   e.g. movements of forehead, eyebrows, periorbital area, cheeks; include frowning, blinking, smiling, grimacing.

   ☐ 0 = None
   1 = Minimal (may be extreme normal)
   2 = Mild
   3 = Moderate
   4 = Severe

2. **Lips and perioral area**
   ☐ e.g. puckering, pouting, smacking.
   0 = None
   1 = Minimal (may be extreme normal)
   2 = Mild
   3 = Moderate
   4 = Severe

3. **Jaw**
   ☐ e.g. biting, clenching, chewing, mouth opening, lateral movements.
   0 = None
   1 = Minimal (may be extreme normal)
   2 = Mild
   3 = Moderate
   4 = Severe

4. **Tongue**
   ☐ Rate only increase in movement both in and out of mouth, **not** inability to sustain movement.
   0 = None
   1 = Minimal (may be extreme normal)
   2 = Mild
   3 = Moderate
   4 = Severe

EXTREMITY MOVEMENTS
5. **Upper (arms, wrists, hands, fingers)**
   Include choreic movements (i.e. rapid, objectively purposeless, irregular, spontaneous) and athetoid movements (i.e. slow, irregular, complex, serpentine). Do **not** include tremor (i.e. repetitive, regular, rhythmic).

   ☐ 0 = None
   1 = Minimal (may be extreme normal)
   2 = Mild
   3 = Moderate
   4 = Severe

6.   **Lower (legs, knees, ankles, toes)**
      e.g. lateral knee movement, foot tapping, heel dropping, foot squirming, inversion and
      eversion of foot.
      0 = None
      1 = Minimal (may be extreme normal)
      2 = Mild
      3 = Moderate
      4 = Severe

TRUNK MOVEMENTS
7.   **Neck, shoulders, hip**
      e.g. rocking, twisting, squirming, pelvic gyrations.
      0 = None
      1 = Minimal (may be extreme normal)
      2 = Mild
      3 = Moderate
      4 = Severe

GLOBAL JUDGEMENTS
8.   **Severity of abnormal movements.**
      0 = None
      1 = Minimal
      2 = Mild
      3 = Moderate
      4 = Severe
9.   **Incapacitation due to abnormal movements.**
      0 = None/normal
      1 = Minimal
      2 = Mild
      3 = Moderate
      4 = Severe
10.   **Patient's awareness of abnormal movements.**
      Rate only patient's report.
      0 = No awareness
      1 = Aware, no distress
      2 = Aware, mild distress
      3 = Aware, moderate distress
      4 = Aware, severe distress

DENTAL STATUS

Any current problems with teeth and/or dentures?	☐ YES	☐ NO
Does patient usually wear dentures?	☐ YES	☐ NO

Reproduced from United States Department of Health Education and Welfare 1985. In: Weiner and Lang (1995) *Neurology of Mental Disorders: Advances in Neurology.* New York: Raven Press.

LUNSERS

Please indicate how much you have experienced each of the following symptoms in **the last month** by ticking the appropriate boxes.

	Not at all	Very little	A little	Quite a lot	Very much
1. Rash	☐	☐	☐	☐	☐
2. Difficulty staying awake during the day	☐	☐	☐	☐	☐
3. Runny nose	☐	☐	☐	☐	☐
4. Increased dreaming	☐	☐	☐	☐	☐
5. Headaches	☐	☐	☐	☐	☐
6. Dry mouth	☐	☐	☐	☐	☐
7. Swollen or tender chest	☐	☐	☐	☐	☐
8. Chilblains	☐	☐	☐	☐	☐
9. Difficulty in concentrating	☐	☐	☐	☐	☐
10. Constipation	☐	☐	☐	☐	☐
11. Hair loss	☐	☐	☐	☐	☐
12. Urine darker than usual	☐	☐	☐	☐	☐
13. Period problems	☐	☐	☐	☐	☐
14. Tension	☐	☐	☐	☐	☐
15. Dizziness	☐	☐	☐	☐	☐
16. Feeling sick	☐	☐	☐	☐	☐
17. Increased sex drive	☐	☐	☐	☐	☐
18. Tiredness	☐	☐	☐	☐	☐
19. Muscle stiffness	☐	☐	☐	☐	☐
20. Palpitations	☐	☐	☐	☐	☐
21. Difficulty in remembering things	☐	☐	☐	☐	☐
22. Losing weight	☐	☐	☐	☐	☐
23. Lack of emotions	☐	☐	☐	☐	☐
24. Difficulty achieving climax	☐	☐	☐	☐	☐
25. Weak fingernails	☐	☐	☐	☐	☐
26. Depression	☐	☐	☐	☐	☐
27. Increased sweating	☐	☐	☐	☐	☐
28. Mouth ulcers	☐	☐	☐	☐	☐
29. Slowing of movements	☐	☐	☐	☐	☐
30. Greasy skin	☐	☐	☐	☐	☐

	Not at all	Very little	A little	Quite a lot	Very much
31. Sleeping too much	☐	☐	☐	☐	☐
32. Difficulty passing water	☐	☐	☐	☐	☐
33. Flushing of face	☐	☐	☐	☐	☐
34. Muscle spasms	☐	☐	☐	☐	☐
35. Sensitivity to sun	☐	☐	☐	☐	☐
36. Diarrhoea	☐	☐	☐	☐	☐
37. Over-wet or drooling mouth	☐	☐	☐	☐	☐
38. Blurred vision	☐	☐	☐	☐	☐
39. Putting on weight	☐	☐	☐	☐	☐
40. Restlessness	☐	☐	☐	☐	☐
41. Difficulty getting to sleep	☐	☐	☐	☐	☐
42. Neck muscles aching	☐	☐	☐	☐	☐
43. Shakiness	☐	☐	☐	☐	☐
44. Pins and needles	☐	☐	☐	☐	☐
45. Painful joints	☐	☐	☐	☐	☐
46. Reduced sex drive	☐	☐	☐	☐	☐
47. New or unusual skin marks	☐	☐	☐	☐	☐
48. Parts of body moving on their own	☐	☐	☐	☐	☐
49. Itchy skin	☐	☐	☐	☐	☐
50. Periods less frequent	☐	☐	☐	☐	☐
51. Passing a lot of water	☐	☐	☐	☐	☐

Reproduced by permission of the Royal College of Psychiatrists from Day et al (1995) *Br J Psychiatry* **166**, 650–3.

Sexual Functioning Questionnaire (SFQ)

Patient No. _____   Date. _____

Each statement is followed by a TRUE or FALSE answer. Read each statement carefully and decide which response best describes how you feel. Then put a circle round the corresponding response. If you are not completely sure which response is more accurate, circle the response that you feel is most appropriate. Please ask the person interviewing you if there are any words you do not understand. Do not spend too long on each statement. It is important that you answer each question as honestly as possible. Remember to answer every question.
ALL INFORMATION WILL BE TREATED WITH THE STRICTEST CONFIDENCE.

Over the past month

1. I have thought about sex

    a. at least once per day . . . . TRUE/FALSE

    b. three times a week . . . . TRUE/FALSE

    c. less than once a week . . . . TRUE/FALSE

    d. less than once a fortnight . . . . TRUE/FALSE

2. I never think about sex . . . . TRUE/FALSE

3. I have found other people sexually desirable . . . . TRUE/FALSE

4. I have not wanted to have sexual intercourse . . . . TRUE/FALSE

5. I have enjoyed sex . . . . TRUE/FALSE

6. I have not been particularly interested in sex . . . . TRUE/FALSE

Over the past month

7. I have been easily aroused sexually . . . . TRUE/FALSE

8. It has taken longer than usual for me to become sexually aroused . . . . TRUE/FALSE

9. I have been completely unable to become sexually aroused . . . . TRUE/FALSE

10. Although I have been aroused mentally, nothing has happened physically . . . . TRUE/FALSE

Please answer the next section only if you are male.

Over the past month

11. I have had erections (morning erections or erections on awaking)

    a. every day . . . . TRUE/FALSE

    b. about three times per week . . . . TRUE/FALSE

    c. less than once a fortnight . . . . TRUE/FALSE

    d. less than once a fortnight . . . . TRUE/FALSE

    e. less than once per month . . . . TRUE/FALSE

12. I do not have erections . . . . TRUE/FALSE

13. I am always able to achieve a full erection if I want to . . . . TRUE/FALSE

14. I feel that my erections are not as full now as they used to be .... TRUE/FALSE

15. I am never able to achieve a full erection .... TRUE/FALSE

16. I rarely achieve a full erection .... TRUE/FALSE

17. Because I cannot achieve a full erection, I am unable to have intercourse ..... TRUE/FALSE

Please answer this next section only if you are female

Over the past month

18. Sex has been difficult or painful for me because I do not respond physically as I ought to .... TRUE/FALSE

19. My physical response to sexual stimulation is different now to what it used to be .... TRUE/FALSE

20. My physical response to sexual stimulation is better now than it used to be ... TRUE/FALSE

21. My physical response to sexual stimulation is worse now than it used to be ... TRUE/FALSE

Over the past month

22. I have masturbated

    a. at least once a day .... TRUE/FALSE

    b. about three times per week .... TRUE/FALSE

    c. about once per week .... TRUE/FALSE

    d. less than once per fortnight .... TRUE/FALSE

    e. less than once per month .... TRUE/FALSE

23. I feel that masturbation is wrong .... TRUE/FALSE

24. I never masturbate .... TRUE/FALSE

25. I rarely masturbate .... TRUE/FALSE

26. I have masturbated more often than I usually do .... TRUE/FALSE

27. I have masturbated less than I usually do .... TRUE/FALSE

Over the past month

28. I have not achieved orgasm/ejaculation by any means at all .... TRUE/FALSE

29. I have had orgasms/ejaculations as often as I have wanted .... TRUE/FALSE

30. I have never had an orgasm/ejaculation .... TRUE/FALSE

31. Orgasm/ejaculation has been painful for me .... TRUE/FALSE

32. My orgasm/ejaculation has been different to before .... TRUE/FALSE

33. I have an orgasm/ejaculate every time I have sex/masturbate .... TRUE/FALSE

Please answer the following if you are male

34. I ejaculate a long time after I have achieved orgasm .... TRUE/FALSE

35. My ejaculation happens too quickly .... TRUE/FALSE

36. The amount of fluid that I produce when I ejaculate is less than I used to produce before . . . . TRUE/FALSE

37. The amount of fluid that I produce when I ejaculate is more than I used to produce before . . . . TRUE/FALSE

38. The colour of the fluid that I produce when I ejaculate is different to before . . TRUE/FALSE

Instructions for Interviewer

A. Although this has the appearance of a structured questionnaire, the nature of the topic often means that you will need to clarify terms in order to ensure that the subjects know what is being asked of them. Also, if you are able to talk about sex, the subjects may feel more comfortable when filling in the questionnaire.

B. Remind the subjects that the questions are quite personal, but also normalise the experience by reminding them of the usual process of sexual intercourse and the problems that people might encounter if their sexual function is poor (e.g. 'Usually in order for people to have sex, they have to have an erection, some people find that they have difficulties with this. Section three asks questions about this area' or 'Some people complain of difficulties with their sex life, they may have problems getting aroused sexually or they can't have orgasms, this questionnaire asks about this kind of thing').

C. Section Two: sexual arousal involves the mental phenomena of being sexually interested and is usually accompanied by penile erection in males and vaginal lubrication and swelling of the vaginal walls in females (usual physical response after sexual stimulation in women).

D. Terms

Erection – when the penis gets hard or stiff.

Vaginal lubrication – when the vagina becomes moist.

Orgasm – the feeling that happens at the end of sex. This is usually accompanied by overwhelming physical sensations in women, along with vaginal wall contractions. In men it is a accompanied by ejaculation.

Ejaculation – the production of seminal fluid or semen.

Reproduced by permission of the Royal College of Psychiatrists from Smith et al (2002) *Br J Psychiatry* **181**, 49–55.

Sexual Dysfunction Checklist

Date

Name

Please tick as appropriate

Symptom	Absent 0	Mild 1	Moderate 2	Severe 3	Not applicable/ assessed
Menorrhagia					
Amenorrhoea					
Galctorrhoea					
Gynaecomastia					
Increased libido					
Decreased libido					
Erectile dysfunction					
Ejaculatory dysfunction					
Orgastic dysfunction					
Dry vagina					
Score:					

Comments:

Reproduced by permission of Blackwell Science from Lingjaerde et al (1987) *Acta Psychiatr Scand* **34** (suppl. 76), 1–100.

Client Service Receipt Inventory

General Version, November 1994

1. Refer to header

Date of interview 1 [| | | 2 | 0 | 0 |]
                              D   M   Y

2. **EMPLOYMENT AND INCOME**

If yes please describe patient's occupation

	Yes		No	

2.1 Is patient usually in open employment? ☐ 2 ☐ 3 _____
Y   N

	Yes	No	

Is patient currently 'off sick'? ☐ 4 ☐
Y   N

If yes: for how many days? 5 [| | |] days (to the nearest half day)

Yes   No

Is patient currently a student? ☐ 6 ☐
Does patient have primary home-making ☐ 7 ☐
responsibilities?
Is patient currently unemployed? ☐ 8 ☐
Y   N

If yes: when was the patient last in 9 [| | | 2 | 0 | 0 |]
employment?   D   M   Y

Yes   No

2.2 Is the patient currently in sheltered ☐ 10 ☐
employment? Y   N

	11
If yes: please tick box which best describes patient's occupation	
Volunteer work	☐ 1
Job training	☐ 2
Sheltered work (permanent)	☐ 3
Sheltered work (rehabilitation)	☐ 4
Clubhouse	☐ 5

Gross wage per week in local currency
(please give estimate if actual amount not known) 12 [| | | | | | |]

Yes   No

2.3 Does the patient currently receive social ☐ 13 ☐
security benefits? Y   N

If yes: amount received per week in local currency
(please give estimate if actual amount not known,
excluding housing benefit) 14 [| | | | | | |]

If amount is not given please list benefits by name
15 [| | | | | | |]

Does the patient have any other source of Yes   No
income, e.g. from relatives, friends or ☐ 16 ☐
information/hidden economy? Y   N

If yes: amount received per week in local currency
(please give estimate if actual amount not known)   17 [| | | | | | | |]

3. ACCOMMODATION

3.1 Postcode/area code for current address   18 [| | | | | | | |]

3.2 When did patient move to the current address? *(✓ one box)*

19

More than 12 months ago   □ 1
3–12 months ago   □ 2
Less than 3 months ago   □ 3

3.3 How many bedrooms are there in the
current accommodation?   20 [| |]

3.4 Patient contribution to current
accommodation per week in local currency
(please give estimate if actual amount not known)   21 [| | | | | | | |]

	Yes		No

3.5 Does the patient live in specialised   □   22   □
accommodation?

If yes: is accommodation only for people   □   23   □
with mental health problems?   Y   N

Is specialised accommodation provided under
any of the following arrangements? *(✓ one box)*

Lodging house	24	□ 1	Warden assisted housing	□ 4
Bed and breakfast		□ 2	Adult fostering arrangements	□ 5
Overnight hostel/shelter		□ 3	Other*	□ 9

* Please specify 25 _____

Staff cover during the day *(✓ one box)*

26

No staff cover   □ 1
Ad hoc staff cover   □ 2
Regular but not continuous staff cover □ 3
Continuous staff cover   □ 4

Staff cover at night *(✓ all relevant boxes)*   27
No staff cover   □ 1
On call staff cover   □ 2
Sleeping staff on premises   □ 4
Waking staff on premises   □ 5

Total number of care staff working in the
facility   28   □
(please give estimate if actual number not known)

Number of residents at this accommodation   29   □
(please give estimate if actual number not known)

Managing agency for this accommodation *(please ✓ and enter name of agency)*

30

Health authority	□ 1	Name of agency
Health trust social services	□ 2	31 _____
Voluntary organisation	□ 3	
Private organisation	□ 4	

		Yes		No
3.6	Does the patient live in domestic accommodation?	□	32	□
		Y		N

If yes: tenure of accommodation (✓ *one box*)

33
Privately rented □ 1
Local authority rented □ 2
Housing association rented □ 3
Owner occupied □ 4   *Please describe
Other* □ 5   34 _____

Total number of adults in accommodation?   35 |__|__|

Total number children below the age of   36 |__|__|
16 inaccommodation?

Please state household income per week in   37 |__|__|__|__|__|__|__|
local currency

4. SERVICE RECEIPT (1)

4.1 Hospital in-patient services used by patient in the previous 3 months
   (please list all admissions)

Name of hospital	No. of days as psychiatric in-patient	No. of days as non-psychiatric in-patient
	38 |__|__|	44 |__|__|
	39 |__|__|	45 |__|__|
	40 |__|__|	46 |__|__|
	41 |__|__|	47 |__|__|
	42 |__|__|	48 |__|__|
	43 |__|__|	49 |__|__|
	44 |__|__|	50 |__|__|
	45 |__|__|	51 |__|__|
	46 |__|__|	52 |__|__|
	47 |__|__|	53 |__|__|
	48 |__|__|	54 |__|__|
	49 |__|__|	55 |__|__|
	50 |__|__|	56 |__|__|
	51 |__|__|	57 |__|__|
	52 |__|__|	58 |__|__|
	53 |__|__|	59 |__|__|
	54 |__|__|	60 |__|__|
	55 |__|__|	61 |__|__|

4.2 Other hospital services used by patient in the previous 3 months

Service attended	No. of psychiatric attendances in previous 3 months	No. of non-psychiatric attendances in previous 3 months
Accident and Emergency	62 ⬚⬚⬚	63 ⬚⬚⬚
Other out-patient	64 ⬚⬚⬚	65 ⬚⬚⬚
Day hospital	66 ⬚⬚⬚	67 ⬚⬚⬚

4.3 Criminal justice services used by patient in the previous 3 months

	Number	Average duration of contact		
		Days	Hours	Minutes
Arrests	68 ⬚⬚⬚	69 ⬚⬚⬚	70 ⬚⬚⬚	71 ⬚⬚⬚
Visits to lawyer	72 ⬚⬚⬚	73 ⬚⬚⬚	74 ⬚⬚⬚	75 ⬚⬚⬚
Court appearances	76 ⬚⬚⬚	77 ⬚⬚⬚	78 ⬚⬚⬚	79 ⬚⬚⬚
Contacts with probation officer	80 ⬚⬚⬚	81 ⬚⬚⬚	82 ⬚⬚⬚	83 ⬚⬚⬚
Contacts with police	84 ⬚⬚⬚	85 ⬚⬚⬚	86 ⬚⬚⬚	87 ⬚⬚⬚
Nights spent in police cell or prison	88 ⬚⬚⬚	89 ⬚⬚⬚	90 ⬚⬚⬚	91 ⬚⬚⬚

4.4 Care-giver time

During the previous 3 months, how many hours care per week *on average* has the patient received from all informal carers on the following tasks?

Tasks	*Average* hours received per week	
	from co-residents	from other friends & relatives
Personal care	92 ⬚⬚⬚	93 ⬚⬚⬚
Providing transport	94 ⬚⬚⬚	95 ⬚⬚⬚
Preparing meals	96 ⬚⬚⬚	97 ⬚⬚⬚
Housework/laundry	98 ⬚⬚⬚	99 ⬚⬚⬚
DIY	100 ⬚⬚⬚	101 ⬚⬚⬚
Gardening	102 ⬚⬚⬚	103 ⬚⬚⬚
Shopping/collecting benefits	104 ⬚⬚⬚	105 ⬚⬚⬚
Arranging meetings	106 ⬚⬚⬚	107 ⬚⬚⬚
Socialising/companionship	108 ⬚⬚⬚	109 ⬚⬚⬚

5. SERVICE RECEIPT (II) – REDUCED LIST METHODOLOGY

5.1 Community services used by patient in the previous 3 months
Number of day care attendances   110 ⬚⬚⬚
(*Note: 1 attendance = a session, i.e. whole of morning or afternoon*)
Name of most commonly used day/drop-in centre   111 _____

Number of times patient has seen a community psychiatric nurse   112 ⬚⬚⬚

Average duration of visit in minutes   113 ⬚⬚⬚ min

Number of times patient has seen a social worker   114 ☐|☐

Average duration of visit in minutes   115 ☐|☐ min

Number of times patient has seen a general practitioner/family physician   116 ☐|☐

Please list other services which patient has used more than once a month in the previous 3 months

117 _____

_____

_____

_____

_____

Developed by Jennifer Beecham and Martin Knapp, University of Kent at Canterbury, Institute of Psychiatry (King's College London) and London School of Economics.

Definitions for Client Service Inventory

1. Refers to Patient Identification which is completed at the top of the form.

Employment & Income

2.1 'Homemaking responsibilities' refers to duties performed, regardless of sex, by mothers with schizophrenia or men with schizophrenia whose main occupation would be to keep the home clean and tidy and perhaps provide shopping and/or meals.

2.2 'Clubhouse' – a user patient-run programme that aims to provide work for its members. Each member aims to take on work for industry or small businesses, etc. Each member is shadowed by a more capable person. The contract with the business is a joint contract which commits the patient and the more capable person to doing the work and therefore providing a guarantee that the work will be completed. The average Club has 50–60 members of which 10–20% will be working at any one time. For the others, the Club provides a social day centre.

Where monthly amounts are usually provided please derive the weekly amount as follows:

$$\frac{\text{monthly total}}{4} = \text{weekly total}$$

3.5 'Voluntary organisation' refers to 'non-profit' organisations, for example a church organisation.
'Private organisation' refers to 'for profit' organisations, for example the organisation has an income by being the managing organisation.

4.2 'A & E attendances' are unplanned visits to the accident and emergency department.
'Other out-patient attendance' is defined as a short visit to medical or paramedical staff within the hospital.
'Day hospital attendance' is where the patient is expected to attend a department or ward for a half or full day and does not include overnight stay. Examples would be minor surgery or industrial therapy.

Drug Attitude Inventory (DAI 10)

1) For me, the good things about medication outweigh the bad
   T   F

2) I feel weird, like a zombie on medication
   T   F

3) I take medication of my own free choice
   T   F

4) Medication makes me feel more relaxed
   T   F

5) Medication makes me feel tired and sluggish
   T   F

6) I take medication only when I am sick
   T   F

7) I feel more normal on medication
   T   F

8) It is unnatural for my mind and body to be controlled on medication
   T   F

9) My thoughts are clearer on medication
   T   F

10) By staying on medication, I can prevent getting sick
    T   F

Reproduced by permission of Cambridge University Press from Hogan et al (1983) *Psychological Med* 13, 177–83.

The UKU Side-effect Rating Scale

1. Psychic side-effects
1.1 Concentration difficulties
Difficulties in ability to concentrate, to collect one's thoughts, or to sustain one's attention.
- 0: No or doubtful difficulties in concentrating.
- 1: The patient must try harder than usual to collect his thoughts, but not to the degree that it hampers the patient in his everyday life.
- 2: The difficulties in concentrating are pronounced enough to hamper the patient in his everyday life.
- 3: The patient's difficulties in concentrating are obvious to the interviewer during the interview.

1.2 Asthenia/lassitude/increased fatiguability
The patient's experience of lassitude and lack of endurance. The assessment is based upon the patient's reported statements.
- 0: No or doubtful lassitude.
- 1: The patient tires more easily than usual; however, this does not mean that the patient needs to rest more than usual during the day.
- 2: Must rest now and then during the day because of lassitude.
- 3: Must rest most of the day because of lassitude.

1.3 Sleepiness/sedation

Diminished ability to stay awake during the day. The assessment is based on clinical signs during the interview.

   0: No or doubtful sleepiness.

   1: Slightly sleepy/drowsy as regards facial expression and speech.

   2: More markedly sleepy/drowsy. The patient yawns and tends to fall asleep when there is a pause in the conversation.

   3: Difficult to keep the patient awake and to wake the patient, respectively.

1.4 Failing memory

Impaired memory. Assessment should be independent of any concentration difficulties.

   0: No or doubtful disturbances of memory.

   1: Slight, subjective feeling of reduced memory compared with the patient's usual condition; however, not interfering with functioning.

   2: The failing memory hampers the patient and/or slight signs of this are observed during the interview.

   3: The patient shows clear signs of failing memory during the interview.

1.5 Depression

Includes both the verbal and the non-verbal expressions of the patient's experience of sadness, depression, melancholy, hopelessness, helplessness, perhaps with suicidal impulses.

   0: Neutral or elated mood.

   1: The patient's mood is somewhat more depressed and sad than usual; however, the patient still finds life worth living.

   2: The patient's mood is clearly depressed, perhaps including non-verbal expressions of hopelessness and/or wishes of dying, but the patient has no direct plans to commit suicide.

   3: The patient's verbal and non-verbal expressions of hopelessness and sadness are great and/or it is considered highly likely that he plans to commit suicide.

1.6 Tension/inner unrest

Inability to relax, nervous restlessness. This item is to be assessed on the basis of the patient's experience and must be distinguished from motor akathisia (Item 2.6).

   0: No or doubtful tension/nervous restlessness.

   1: The patient states that he is slightly tense and restless; however, this does not interfere with his functioning.

   2: Considerable tension and inner unrest; however, without this being so intense or constant that the patient's daily life is influenced to any marked degree.

   3: The patient feels tension or restlessness that is so marked that his daily life is clearly affected.

1.7 Increased duration of sleep

This should be assessed on the basis of the average of sleep over the three preceding nights. The assessment is to be made in relation to the patient's usual pre-illness state.

   0: No or doubtful increase of the duration of sleep.

   1: Sleeps up to 2 hours longer than usual.

   2: Sleeps 2 or 3 hours longer than usual.

   3: Sleeps more than 3 hours longer than usual.

1.8 Reduced duration of sleep

Should be assessed on the basis of the average of sleep over the three preceding nights. The assessment is to be made in relation to the patient's usual pre-illness state.

   0: No or doubtful reduction of the duration of sleep.

   1: Sleeps up to 2 hours less than usual.

   2: Sleeps 2 or 3 hours less than usual.

   3: Sleeps more than 3 hours less than usual.

1.9 Increased dream activity
Should be assessed independently of dream content and based on the average of sleep over the three preceding nights in relation to the usual pre-illness dream activity.

   0: No or doubtful change in the dream activity.
   1: Slightly increased dream activity, which does not disturb the night's sleep, however.
   2: More pronounced increase of dream activity.
   3: Very pronounced increase of dream activity.

1.10 Emotional indifference
A diminution of the patient's empathy, leading to apathy.

   0: No or doubtful emotional indifference.
   1: Slight subduing of the patient's empathy.
   2: Obvious emotional indifference.
   3: Pronounced indifference so that the patient behaves apathetically in relation to his surroundings.

2. Neurological side-effects

2.1 Dystonia
Acute forms of dystonia in the form of tonic muscular contractions localized to one or several muscle groups, particularly in the mouth, tongue, and/or neck. The assessment is to be made on the basis of the last three days preceding the examination.

   0: No or doubtful dystonia.
   1: Very slight or short spasms, for instance in the musculature of the jaws or the neck.
   2: More pronounced contractions of a longer duration and/or of a wider localization.
   3: Marked forms of for instance oculogyric crises or opisthotonus.

2.2 Rigidity
Increased muscle tone of a uniform and general nature, observed on the basis of a uniform, steady resistance to passive movements of the limbs. Special importance is attached to the muscles around the elbow joints and shoulders.

   0: No or doubtful rigidity.
   1: Slight rigidity in neck, shoulder, and extremities. It must be possible to observe the rigidity on the basis of resistance to passive movements of the elbow joints.
   2: Medium rigidity assessed on the basis of resistance to passive movements of for instance the elbow joints.
   3: Very marked rigidity.

2.3 Hypokinesia/akinesia
Slow movements (bradykinesia), reduced facial expression, reduced arm swinging, reduced length of stride, perhaps leading to cessation of movement (akinesia).

   0: No or doubtful hypokinesia
   1: Slightly reduced movement, for instance slightly reduced swinging of an arm when walking or slightly reduced facial expressions.
   2: More clear reduction of mobility, for instance slow walking.
   3: Very marked reduction of mobility, bordering on and including akinesia, e.g. parkinsonian mask and/or very short length of stride.

2.4 Hyperkinesia
Involuntary movements, most frequently affecting the oro-facial region in the form of the so-called bucco-linguo-masticatory syndrome. However, it is often also seen in the extremities, especially the fingers, more rarely in the musculature of the body and the respiratory system. Both initial and tardive hyperkinesias are included.

   0: No or doubtful hyperkinesia.
   1: Slight hyperkinesia, only present intermittently.
   2: Moderate hyperkinesia, present most of the time.
   3: Severe hyperkinesia, present most of the time, with for instance marked tongue protrusion, opening of the mouth, facial hyperkinesia, with or without involvement of the extremities.

2.5 Tremor

This item comprises all forms of tremor.

- 0: No or doubtful tremor.
- 1: Very slight tremor that does not hamper the patient.
- 2: Clear tremor hampering the patient, the amplitude of finger tremor being less than 3 cm.
- 3: Clear tremor with an amplitude of more than 3 cm and which cannot be controlled by the patient.

2.6 Akathisia

A subjective feeling and objective signs of muscle unrest, particularly in the lower extremities, so that it may be difficult for the patient to remain seated. Assessment of this item is based on clinical signs observed during the interview, as well as on the patient's report.

- 0: No or doubtful akathisia.
- 1: Slight akathisia; however, the patient can keep still without effort.
- 2: Moderate akathisia; however, the patient can, with an effort, remain sitting during the interview.
- 3: When the patient has to rise to his feet several times during the interview because of akathisia.

2.7 Epileptic seizures

- 0: No seizures within the last 6 months.
- 1: One single seizure within the last 6 months.
- 2: 2 or 3 seizures within the last 6 months.
- 3: More than 3 seizures within the last 6 months.

2.8 Paraesthesias

Pricking, creeping, or burning sensations in the skin.

- 0: No or doubtful paraesthesias.
- 1: Mild paraesthesias, scarcely bothering the patient.
- 2: Moderate paraesthesias, clearly bothering the patient.
- 3: Severe paraesthesias, markedly bothering the patient.

3. Autonomic side-effects

3.1 Accommodation disturbances

Difficulty in seeing clearly or distinctly at close quarters (with or without glasses), whereas the patient sees clearly at a long distance. If the patient uses bifocal glasses, the condition must be assessed on the basis of the use of the distance glasses.

- 0: No difficulty in reading an ordinary newspaper text.
- 1: Newspaper text can be read, but the patient's eyes tire rapidly and/or he must hold the paper further away.
- 2: The patient cannot read an ordinary newspaper text, but still manages to read texts printed in larger types.
- 3: The patient can read large type, such as a headline, only with aid, such as magnifying glass.

3.2 Increased salivation

Increased, non-stimulated salivation.

- 0: No or doubtful increase of salivation.
- 1: Salivation clearly increased, but not bothersome.
- 2: Disturbing increase of salivation; need for spitting or frequent swallowing of saliva; only exceptional dribbling.
- 3: Frequent or constant dribbling, perhaps concomitant speech disturbances.

3.3 Reduced salivation (dryness of mouth)

Dryness of mouth because of diminished salivation. May result in increased consumption of liquids, but must be distinguished from thirst.

- 0: No or doubtful dryness of mouth.
- 1: Slight dryness of mouth, not disturbing to the patient.
- 2: Moderate and slightly disturbing dryness of mouth.
- 3: Marked dryness of mouth which clearly disturbs the patient's daily life.

3.4 Nausea/vomiting

To be recorded on the basis of the last 3 days.

 0: No or doubtful nausea.
 1: Slight nausea.
 2: Disturbing nausea, but without vomiting.
 3: Nausea with vomiting.

3.5 Diarrhoea

Increased frequency and/or thinner consistency of faeces.

 0: No or doubtful diarrhoea.
 1: Clearly present, but does not disturb work or other performance.
 2: Disturbing, with need for several daily, inconvenient stools.
 3: Marked, imperative need for defaecation, threatening or actual incontinence, results in frequent interruptions of work.

3.6 Constipation

Reduced frequency of defaecation and/or thicker consistency of faeces.

 0: No or doubtful constipation.
 1: Slight constipation, but bearable.
 2: More marked constipation which hampers the patient.
 3: Very pronounced constipation.

3.7 Micturition disturbances

Feeling of difficulty in starting and of resistance to micturition, weaker stream and/or increased time of micturition. Should be assessed on the basis of the last 3 days.

 0: No or doubtful micturition disturbances.
 1: Clearly present, but bearable.
 2: Poor stream, considerably increased time of micturition, feeling of incomplete emptying of bladder.
 3: Retention of urine with high-volume residual urine and/or threatened or actual acute retention.

3.8 Polyuria/polydipsia

Increased urine production resulting in increased frequency of micturition and discharge of an abundant quantity of urine at each micturition; secondarily increased consumption of fluid.

 0: No or doubtful.
 1: Clearly present, but not hampering. Nocturia: at most once a night (in young people).
 2: Moderately hampering because of frequent thirst, nocturia two or three times a night, or micturition more frequent than every two hours.
 3: Very hampering, almost constant thirst, nocturia at least four times a night, or micturition at least every hour.

3.9 Orthostatic dizziness

Feeling of weakness, everything going black, buzzing in the ears, increasing tendency to faint when changing from supine or sitting position to upright position.

 0: No or doubtful.
 1: Clearly present, but requires no special countermeasures.
 2: Hampering, but can be neutralized by slow and/or stagewise change to upright position.
 3: Threatening fainting or real episodes of fainting despite careful change of position, with a tendency to this type of dizziness as long as the patient is in an upright position.

3.10 Palpitations/tachycardia

Palpitation, feeling of rapid, strong and/or irregular heartbeats.

 0: No or doubtful.
 1: Clearly present, but not hampering, only short occasional attacks or more constant, but not marked palpitation.
 2: Hampering frequent or constant palpitation that worries the patient or disturbs his night's sleep; however, without concomitant symptoms.

3: Suspicion of real tachycardia, for instance because of concomitant feeling of weakness and need to lie down, dyspnoea, tendency to fainting, or precordial pain.

3.11 Increased tendency to sweating

Localized to the whole body, not only palms and soles of the feet.

0: No or doubtful.
1: Clearly present, but mild, for example a profuse outburst of sweat only after considerable effort.
2: Hampering, requires frequent change of clothes, profuse sweating after moderate activity, for instance walking up stairs.
3: Profuse outbursts of sweat after slight activity or when resting; the patient is constantly wet, must change clothes several times a day and must also change night clothes and/or bedclothes.

4. Other side-effects

4.1 Rash

On the scoring sheet the type of rash is classified as a) morbilliform, b) petechial, c) urticarial, d) psoriatic, and e) cannot be classified. The following grading is used:

0: No or doubtful rash.
1: Localized to less than 5 per cent of the skin surface, for instance to the palms.
2: Scattered all over the skin, but covers less than 1/3 of the skin surface.
3: Universal, i.e. covers more than 1/3 of the skin surface.

4.2 Pruritus

0: No or doubtful.
1: Slight pruritus.
2: Pronounced pruritus, so that the patient is being hampered. There may be scratch marks.
3: Severe pruritus that markedly hampers the patient. There are distinct skin changes because of scratching.

4.3 Photosensitivity

Increased sensitivity to sunlight.

0: No or doubtful.
1: Slight, but not hampering.
2: More pronounced and hampering to the patient.
3: So pronounced that drug withdrawal is clearly necessary.

4.4 Increased pigmentation

Increased skin pigmentation of brown or other colour, often localized to parts of the skin exposed to light.

0: No or doubtful increase of pigmentation.
1: Slightly increased pigmentation.
2: Such marked pigmentation, generally or localized, that it worries the patient but is not conspicuous to others.
3: So pronounced that the pigmentation can easily be observed by other people.

4.5 Weight gain

The rating is to be made on the basis of the preceding month.

0: No or doubtful weight gain during the preceding month.
1: Weight gain amounting to 1–2 kg during the preceding month.
2: Weight gain amounting to 3–4 kg during the preceding month.
3: Weight gain amounting to more than 4 kg during the preceding month.

4.6 Weight loss

0: No or doubtful weight loss.
1: Weight loss amounting to 1–2 kg during the preceding month.
2: Weight loss amounting to 3–4 kg during the preceding month.
3: Weight loss amounting to more than 4 kg during the preceding month.

4.7 Menorrhagia

Hypermenorrhoea, polymenorrhoea, or metrorrhagia during the last 3 months.

0: No or doubtful increase in frequency or intensity of menstrual flow.

1: Hypermenorrhoea, i.e. the menstrual flow is more intense than usual, the intervals being normal.
2: Polymenorrhoea, i.e. the menstrual flow occurs more frequently and is more intense than normal.
3: Metrorrhagia, i.e. irregular intervals and intensity, the blood loss being more frequent and intense compared with the usual pattern.

4.8 Amenorrhoea
Hypomenorrhoea, oligomenorrhoea, or amenorrhoea during the last 3 months.
0: No or doubtful reduction in frequency or intensity of menstrual flow.
1: Hypomenorrhoea, i.e. uterine bleeding of less than the normal amount, but occurring at normal intervals.
2: Oligomenorrhoea, i.e. prolonged intervals compared with the usual condition; the intensity may also be lower than usual.
3: Amenorrhoea, i.e. menstruation has been absent for more than 3 months.

4.9 Galactorrhoea
Increased secretion of milk outside periods of breast feeding.
0: No galactorrhoea.
1: Galactorrhoea present, but to a very slight degree.
2: Galactorrhoea is present to a moderate degree and is felt to be somewhat disturbing.
3: Galactorrhoea is very pronounced and clearly disturbing.

4.10 Gynaecomastia
Excessive development of the male mammary glands.
0: No gynaecomastia.
1: Gynaecomastia present to a very slight degree compared with the usual state.
2: Gynaecomastia clearly present; however, only hampering when the patient is undressed.
3: Gynaecomastia present to such a severe degree that it affects the patient cosmetically, as it can be observed even if he is dressed.

4.11 Increased sexual desire
Increased desire for sexual activity.
0: No or doubtful.
1: Slight increase, which is, however, still felt as natural by the partner.
2: Clear increase that has given rise to comments and discussions with the partner.
3: When the usual desire has increased to such a severe extent that the patient's life with his partner is considerably disturbed.

4.12 Diminished sexual desire
Reduced desire for sexual activity.
0: No or doubtful.
1: The desire for sexual activity is slightly diminished, but without hampering the patient.
2: A distinct reduction of the patient's desire for and interest in sexual activities so that it becomes a problem for the patient.
3: Desire and interest have diminished to such an extent that sexual intercourse occurs extremely seldom or has stopped.

4.13 Erectile dysfunction
Difficulty in attaining or maintaining an erection.
0: No or doubtful.
1: Slightly diminished ability to attain or maintain an erection.
2: A distinct change in the patient's ability to attain or maintain an erection.
3: The patient only rarely (or never) can attain or maintain an erection.

4.14 Ejaculatory dysfunction
Dysfunction of the patient's ability to control ejaculation. Includes a) premature or b) delayed ejaculation. On the scoring sheet it should be indicated whether a) or b) is present.
0: No or doubtful.

1: It is somewhat more difficult than usual for the patient to control ejaculation, but it does not trouble him.

2: A distinct change in the patient's ability to control ejaculation, so that it becomes a problem for him.

3: The patient's ability to control ejaculation is influenced to such an extent that it has become a dominating problem in his sexual intercourse and thus to a great extent influences his experience of orgasm.

4.15 Orgastic dysfunction

Difficulty in obtaining and experiencing satisfactory orgasm.

0: No or doubtful.

1: It is more difficult for the patient than usual to obtain orgasm and/or the experience of orgasm is slightly influenced.

2: The patient states that there is a clear change in the ability to obtain orgasm and/or in the experience of orgasm. This change has reached such a degree that it troubles the patient.

3: When the patient rarely or never can obtain orgasm and/or the experience of orgasm is markedly reduced.

4.16 Dry vagina

Dryness of vagina with sexual stimulation.

0: No or doubtful.

1: Slight dryness of vagina with sexual stimulation.

2: Moderately disturbing dryness of vagina with sexual stimulation.

3: Severely disturbing, marked dryness of vagina making coitus difficult (or necessitating the use of lubricants).

4.17 Headache

On the scoring sheet headache is classified as: a) tension headache, b) migraine, c) other forms of headache.

0: No or doubtful headache.

1: Slight headache.

2: Moderate, hampering headache which does not interfere with the patient's daily life.

3: Pronounced headache interfering with the patient's daily life.

4.18 Physical dependence

Appearance of vegetative and/or other somatic symptoms after discontinuation of the drug in question, based on the condition during the last 3 months. Can be assessed only when an attempt has been made to discontinue the drug (indicate the responsible drug on the form).

0: Nothing suggests physical dependence.

1: After discontinuation there were slight vegetative symptoms like tachycardia or an increased tendency to sweating.

2: After discontinuation there were moderate to marked vegetative symptoms and anxiety or restlessness.

3: After discontinuation there were severe vegetative symptoms, anxiety, restlessness and/or convulsions.

4.19 Psychic dependence

Psychic dependence is defined as a strong wish to continue taking the drug because of its psychic effects (or the effects which the patient thinks it has) when these effects are regarded by the doctor as being unwanted or at least unnecessary. Rating should be based on the condition during the last 3 months.

0: No or doubtful psychic dependence.

1: Slight, but not serious psychic dependence.

2: Clear psychic dependence, but without medical or social complications.

3: Pronounced psychic dependence with an almost compulsory wish to continue taking the drug at any price. The use of the drug in question may have caused medical or social complications.

The UKU Side-effect Rating Scale *contd*

TICK APPROPRIATE BOX (DEGREE <u>AND</u> CAUSAL RELATIONSHIP) FOR EACH ITEM

Category of side-effects		Symptom	Not ass.	Degree last 3 days (see manual)				Causal relationship*		
			9	0	1	2	3	imp	pos	prb
Psychic	1.1	Concentration difficulties								
	1.2	Asthenia/lassitude/increased fatiguability								
	1.3	Sleepiness/sedation								
	1.4	Failing memory								
	1.5	Depression								
	1.6	Tension/inner unrest								
	1.7	Increased duration of sleep								
	1.8	Reduced duration of sleep								
	1.9	Increased dream activity								
	1.10	Emotional indifference								
Neurologic	2.1	Dystonia								
	2.2	Rigidity								
	2.3	Hypokinesia/akinesia								
	2.4	Hyperkinesia								
	2.5	Tremor								
	2.6	Akathisia								
	2.7	Epileptic seizures								
	2.8	Paraesthesias								
Autonomic	3.1	Accommodation disturbances								
	3.2	Increased salivation								
	3.3	Reduced salivation								
	3.4	Nausea/vomiting								
	3.5	Diarrhoea								
	3.6	Constipation								
	3.7	Micturition disturbances								
	3.8	Polyuria/polydipsia								
	3.9	Orthostatic dizziness								
	3.10	Palpitations/tachycardia								
	3.11	Increased tendency to sweating								
Other	4.1	Rash								
	4.1a	– Morbilliform								
	4.1b	– Petechial								
	4.1c	– Urticarial								
	4.1d	– Psoriatic								
	4.1e	– Cannot be classified								
	4.2	Pruritus								
	4.3	Photosensitivity								
	4.4	Increased pigmentation								
	4.5	Weight gain								
	4.6	Weight loss								
	4.7	Menorrhagia								
	4.8	Amenorrhoea								
	4.9	Galactorrhoea								

Category of side-effects	Symptom	Not ass.	Degree last 3 days (see manual)				Causal relationship*		
		9	0	1	2	3	imp	pos	prb
Other	4.10 Gynaecomastia								
	4.11 Increased sexual desire								
	4.12 Diminished sexual desire								
	4.13 Erectile dysfunction								
	4.14 Ejaculatory dysfunction								
	4.15 Orgastic dysfunction								
	4.16 Dry vagina								
	4.17 Headache								
	4.17a – Tension headache								
	4.17b – Migraine								
	4.17c – Other forms								
	4.18 Physical dependence								
	4.19 Psychic dependence								

* imp = improbable, pos = possible, prb = probable

Global assessment of the interference by existing side-effects with the patient's <u>daily performance</u>:

		Assessed by	
		Patient	Doctor
0	No side-effects		
1	Mild side-effects that do not interfere with the patient's performance		
2	Side-effects that interfere moderately with the patient's performance		
3	Side-effects that interfere markedly with the patient's performance		

Consequence:

0	No action	
1	More frequent assessment of the patient, but no reduction of dose, and/or occasional drug treatment of side-effects	
2	Reduction of dose and/or continuous drug treatment of side-effects	
3	Discontinuation of drug or change to another preparation	

Date | Day Mth Year | Signature: _____

Reproduced by permission of Blackwell Science from Lingjaerde et al (1987) *Acta Psychiatr Scand* **34** (suppl. 76), 1–100.

Appendix III: A formal guide to taking a psychiatric history

History of presenting complaint

- Why have you come here today / what seems to be the trouble?

- Is there anything else bothering you?

- Whose idea was it to come here?

- Why today? Why not two weeks ago/two weeks from now?

- When did problems begin?

- Any triggers?

- Course since inception – intermittent/constant

- Frequency, duration, severity of symptoms

- Have you ever had anything like this before?

- If so, when / what happened then?

- Is this the worst ever / if not, when was?

Family history

- Parents – age / where born

- Alive / well / sick / what's the trouble

- Dead / when / what of / age when died

- Patient's age when parent(s) died / if recent or in childhood explore further / was death sudden / how did they react / did they attend funeral / is there a gravestone/memorial – do they visit it

- If parents alive, are they still together

- If not or if one parent dead, any new partner on the scene

- Sibs: age, sex, whether biological, marital status, occupation

- Where do they live / is there contact with patient / what is relationship like with patient

- Are sibs in good health / if any dead, how and when

- Was patient a twin

- What was patient's birth rank

Personal history

- Where were you born / what city, country / in hospital or at home

- Was it a normal birth

- Were milestones normal

- Would you describe childhood as happy/sad/bit of both – (elaborate if necessary)

- Did you live at home with parents / if not why / with other relatives / in care – if so, why / what was that like / were you bullied / abused

- How was school / how many schools did you go to (primary and secondary) / did you like it / did you have friends / play truant / get expelled / get bullied or bully / did you do well / when did you leave school / what exams did you attain / were your results good

- Further education: did you have any / what sort / what results / what qualifications

Psychosexual history

- For females: have you ever been pregnant / how many times

- For both: how many children (age, sex) / where do they live / did or do they cause or have problems / how is your relationship with them / are they all right / if they have left home, how much contact is there

- For both: are you married / in relationship / how long for / any serious relationships before this one / if so, who ended them / when did you meet present partner / any separations in this relationship / if so why / any violence / if so, does partner drink/take drugs / what's the worst thing they've ever done to you

- How do you get on / is partner supportive/understanding

Social/work history/circumstances

✦ Longest job ever / what was it / how long for / why did you leave / ever been sacked (what for)

✦ Current job / what is it / how long there / do you like it / do you get on all right with people there / what's your sick leave record like / when did you last go to work

✦ Where are you living / is it owned / rented / council / how many bedrooms / what is it like / what floor is it on (if flat) / are the conditions (heating, etc.) adequate / how long have you been there / who else lives there

✦ Any debts / any creditors after you

✦ Do you have friends / any close friends / people you can confide in / do you maintain contact with them

✦ How do you spend your time / any hobbies

Habits/addictions

✦ Alcohol / do you drink it / how much / if a lot or ever caused you problems (if so, do a full alcohol history)

✦ Any drugs (go through list marijuana, ecstasy, coke, crack, speed, heroin, LSD, pills, etc.)

✦ If takes drugs: do you ever inject them / ever share needles / ever been tested for HIV/ hepatitis / if so, have you used dirty needles / shared needles since last test

✦ If using any drugs: when did you first use / when did you last use / how much do you get through in a week

✦ If stopped but used to: when using were you ever a regular or heavy user

Forensic history

✦ Ever been in trouble with the police / ever been in prison / when / how long for / what's the worst thing you've ever been charged with (even if charges weren't upheld) / ever been charged with GBH or ABH / what's the worst thing you've ever done / ever carried weapons / do you carry them now / any court cases pending / are you on parole

Past psychiatric history

+ When did you first see a psychiatrist / ever admitted to hospital / if so, when and where, for how long, what for, what was treatment / ever been Sectioned

+ If currently seeing psychiatrist, how often / who is it / where / do you attend your appointments / last one / next one

Past medical history

+ Any operations / ever been to hospital for medical things / ever been to Outpatients or A&E / any serious illnesses / head injury /fits

+ Are you on any medication / what for / do you take it / does it help / in what way does it help / who put you on it

+ Any allergies

+ Ever had 'nerve tablets' / did you take them / did they help (if so, how) / why did you stop taking them / how long on them

Mental state examination

Appearance and behaviour

+ Kempt / unkempt (if so, malodorous? Smell of alcohol?)

+ Does patient look stated age? Younger? Older?

+ Reliable historian?

+ Withdrawn / retarded / tearful / agitated / aroused / restless / anxious / suspicious / perplexed / distracted / irritable

+ Rapport / eye contact

+ Mannerisms / abnormal gestures

+ Any evidence of responding to hallucinations / delusions

Speech

+ Amount / rate / flow / volume / animation

+ Answers absent or delayed?

+ Evasive/guarded?

+ Evidence of thought disorder?

Affect

+ Subjective and objective

+ Suicidal ideation (passive/active) or intent?

+ Incongruous affect / lability?

Thoughts

+ Evidence of obsessions/preoccupations

+ Abnormalities of mode of thinking (abnormal perceptions / hallucinations / delusions / abnormal beliefs / overvalued ideas – subculturally acceptable?)

+ Cognition (generally test for gross abnormalities only at this stage)

Cognition

+ Orientation / concentration / attention

Insight/judgement

✦ Awareness of illness

✦ Awareness of help-seeking behaviour

✦ Does patient believe they need psychiatric help/care?

Key references

Addington D, Addington J, Maticka-Tyndale E (1993) Assessing depression in schizophrenia: the Calgary Depression Scale. *Br J Psychiatry* **22** (Suppl.), 39–44.

Allison DB, Mentore JL, Moonseong H et al (1999) Antipsychotic induced weight gain: a comprehensive research synthesis. *Am J Psychiatry* **156**, 1686–96.

Andreasen NC (1982) Negative symptoms in schizophrenia. *Arch Gen Psychiatry* **39**, 784–88.

Atkins JB, Chlan-Fourney J, Nye HE et al (1999) Region specific induction of deltaFosB by repeated administration of typical vs atypical antipsychotic drugs. *Synapse* **33**, 118–28.

Barnes TRE (1989) A rating scale for drug-induced akathisia. *Br J Psychiatry* **154**, 672–76.

Beecham J, Knapp M. (1992) Costing psychiatric interventions. In G Thornicroft, C Brewin, and J Wing (Eds) *Measuring Mental Health Needs*. London: Gaskell pp.163–83.

Bigliani V, Mulligan RS, Acton PD et al (1999) In vivo occupancy of striatal and temporal cortical D2/D3 dopamine receptors by typical antipsychotic drugs – a [123I] epidepride single photon emission tomography (SPET) study. *Br J Psychiatry* **175**, 231–38.

Bigliani V, Mulligan RS, Acton PD et al (2000) Striatal and temporal cortical D2/D3 receptor occupancy by olanzapine – a 123I epidepride single photon emission tomography (SPET) study. *Psychopharmacolog* **150**, 132–40.

Byrom B, Garratt C, Kilpatrick A (1998) Influence of antipsychotic profile on cost of treatment of schizophrenia: A decision analysis approach. *Int J Psych Clin Prac* **2**, 129–38.

Coward DM, Imperato A, Urwyler S et al, (1989) Biochemical and behavioural properties of clozapine. *Psychopharmacology* **99**, S6–S12

Day JC, Wood G, Dewey M, Bentall R (1995) A self-rating scale for measuring neuroleptic side-effects. Validation in a group of schizophrenic patients. *B J Psychiatry* **166**, 650–53.

Duggan L, Fenton M, Dardennes RM et al (2000) Olanzapine for schizophrenia (Cochrane Review). In: *The Cochrane Library*, Issue 1. Oxford: Update Software.

Endicott J, Spitzer RL, Fleiss JL, Cohen J (1976) The global assessment scale. A procedure for measuring overall severity of psychiatric disturbance. *Arch Gen Psychiatry* **33**, 766–71.

Folstein M, Folstein, S, McHugh P (1975) Mini mental state: a practical method for grading the cognitive state of patients for the clinician. *J Psychiatr Res* **12**, 189–98.

Fontaine KR, Moonseong H, Harrigan EP et al (2001) Estimating the consequences of anti-psychotic induced weight gain on health and mortality rate. *Am J Psychiatry* **101**, 277–88.

Gefvert O, Bergstrom M, Langstrom B et al (1998) Time course of central nervous dopamine-D2 and 5-HT2 receptor blockade and plasma drug concentrations after discontinuation of quetiapine (Seroquel) in patients with schizophrenia. *Psychopharmacology* **135**, 119–26.

Goff DC, Henderson DC, Amico E (1992) Cigarette smoking in schizophrenia: relationship to psychopathology and medication side-effects. *Am J Psychiatry* **149**, 1189–94.

Guy W (1976) Assessment Manual for Psychopharmacology Revised. US Dept of Health Education and Welfare, Public Health Service, Alcohol, Drug Abuse and Mental Health Administration, Rockville MD, NIMH pp.218–22.

Haupt DW, Newcomer JW (2001) Hyperglycemia and antipsychotic medications. *J Clin Psychiatry* **62**(suppl 27), 15–26.

Henderson DC, Cagliero E, Gray C et al (2000) Clozapine, diabetes mellitus, weight gain, and lipid abnormalities: A five-year naturalistic study. *Am J Psychiatry* **157**, 975–81.

Hogan TP, Awad AG, Eastwood R (1983) A self-report scale predictive of drug compliance in schizophrenics: reliability and discriminative validity. *Psychological Med* **13**, 177–83.

Kapur S, Zipursky R, Remington G (1999) Clinical and theoretical implications of 5-HT2 and D2 receptor occupancy of clozapine, risperidone, and olanzapine in schizophrenia. *Am J Psychiatry* **156**, 286–93.

Kapur S, Zipursky, Roy P, Jones C, Remington G, Reed K, Houle S (1997) The relationship between D2 receptor occupancy and plasma levels on low dose oral haloperidol: a PET study. *Psychopharmacology* (Berlin) **131**(2), 148–52.

Kapur S, Zipursky R, Jones C et al (2000a) A positron emission tomography study of quetiapine in schizophrenia: a preliminary finding of an antipsychotic effect with only transiently high dopamine D2 receptor occupancy. *Arch Gen Psychiatry* **57**, 553–9.

Kapur S, Zipursky R, Jones C et al (2000b) Relationship between dopamine D(2) occupancy, clinical response, and side-effects: a double-blind PET study of first-episode schizophrenia. *Am J Psychiatry* **157**, 514–20.

Kay SR, Fisbein A, Opler LA (1987) The Positive and Negative Symptom Scale in Schizophrenia. *Schizophrenia Bull* **13**, 261–76.

Kennedy E, Song F, Hunter R et al (2000) Risperidone versus typical antipsychotic medication for schizophrenia (Cochrane Review). In: *The Cochrane Library*, Issue 3, Oxford: Update Software.

Kerwin RW (1994) The New Atypical Antipsychotics. *Br J Psychiatry* **164**, 141–48.

Leucht S, Pitschel-Walz G, Engel RR, Kissling W (2002) Amisulpride, an unusual 'atypical' antipsychotic: a meta-analysis of randomized controlled trials. *Am J Psychiatry* **159**, 180–90.

Levine S (1999) How should we treat extrapyramidal symptoms (EPS)? Clear Perspectives: *Management Issues in Schizophrenia* **1**(2):5–8.

Levinson DF, Simpson GM, Singh H et al (1990) Fluphenazine dose, clinical response, and extrapyramidal symptoms during acute treatment. *Arch Gen Psychiatry* **47**, 761–68.

Lidow MS, Williams GV, Goldman-Rakic PS (1998) The cerebral cortex: a case for a common site of action of antipsychotics. *Trends Pharmacol Sci* **19**, 136–40.

Lingjaerde O, Ahifors U, Bech P et al (1987) The UKU side-effect rating scale. *Acta Psychiatr Scand* **34** (Suppl.) **76**, 1–100.

McEvoy JP, Hogarty GE, Steingard S (1991) Optimal dose of neuroleptic in acute schizophrenia: a controlled study of the neuroleptic threshold and higher haloperidol dose, *Arch Gen Psychiatry* **48**, 739–45.

Meltzer H, Okayli G (1995) Reduction of suicidality during clozapine treatment of neuroleptic-resistant schizophrenia: impact on risk-benefit assessment. *Am J Psychiatry* **152**, 183–90.

Meltzer HY, Matsubara S (1989) The ratios of serotonin and dopamine2 affinities differentiate atypical and typical antipsychotic drugs. *Psychopharmacol Bull* **25**, 390–97.

Mir S, Taylor D (2001) Atypical antipsychotics and hyperglycaemia. *Int Clin Psychopharmacol* **16**, 63–73.

Moore H, West AR, Grace AA (1999) The regulation of forebrain dopamine transmission: relevance to the pathophysiology and psychopathology of schizophrenia. *Biol Psychiatry* **46**, 40–55.

Moore NA, Calligaro DO, Wong DT et al (1993) The pharmacology of olanzapine and other new antipsychotic agents. *Curr Opin Invest Drugs* **2**, 281–93.

Muscoletta G, Barbato G, Pampallona S et al (1999) Extrapyramidal syndromes in neuroleptic treated patients: prevalence, risk factors, and association with tardive dyskinesia. *J Clin Psychopharmacol* **19**, 203–8.

Naber D (1995) A self rating scale to measure subjective effects of neuroleptic drugs, relationships to objective psychopathology, quality of life, compliance and other clinical variables. *Int Clin Psychopharmacol* **10** (suppl. 3), 133–38.

Nasrallah HA, Mulvihill T (2001) Iatrogenic disorders associated with conventional vs typical antipsychotics. *Ann Clin Psychiatry* **13**, 215–27.

Norman RMG, Malla AK, McLean T et al (2000) The relationship of symptoms and level of functioning in schizophrenia to general well-being and the Quality of Life scale. *Acta Psychiatr Scand* **102**, 303–9.

Oakly NR, Hayes AG, Sheehan MJ (1991) Effect of typical and atypical neuroleptics on the behavioural consequences of activation by muscimol of mesolimbic and nigro-striatal dopaminergic pathways in the rat. *Psychopharmacology* **105**, 204–8.

Oosthuizen P, Emsley R, Turner J, Keyter N (2001) Determining the optimal dose of haloperidol in first episode psychosis. *J Psychopharmacol* **15**, 251–55.

Overall JE, Gorham DE (1962) The Brief Psychiatric Rating Scale. *Psychological Reports* **10**, 799–812.

Pilowsky LS, Mulligan RS, Acton PD et al (1997) Limbic selectivity of clozapine. *Lancet* **350**, 490–1.

Rifkin A, Doddi S, Karajgi B et al (1991) Dosage of haloperidol for schizophrenia. *Arch Gen Psychiatry* **48**, 166–70.

Robertson GS, Fibiger HC (1991) Neuroleptics increase *c-fos* expression in the forebrain: contrasting effects of haloperidol and clozapine. *Neuroscience* **46**, 315–28.

Robinson D, Woerner MG, Alvir JM et al (1999). Predictors of relapse following response from a first episode of schizophrenia or schizoaffective disorder. *Arch Gen Psychiatry* 1999 **56**, 241–7.

Seeger TF, Seymour PA, Schmidt AW et al (1995) Ziprasidone (CP-88,059): A new antipsychotic with combined dopamine and srotonin receptor antagonist activity. *J Pharmacol Exp Ther* **275**, 101–13.

Sernyak MJ, Leslie DL, Alarcon RD et al (2002) Association of diabetes mellitus with the use of atypical neuroleptics in the treatment of schizophrenia. *Am J Psychiatry* **159**, 561–66.

Simpson GM, Angus JWS (1970) A rating scale for extra pyramidal side-effects. *Acta Psychiatr Scand* **212**(suppl.), 11–19.

Smith SM, O'Keane V, Murray R (2002). Sexual dysfunction in patients taking conventional antipsychotic medication. *Br J Psychiatry* **181**, 49–55.

Srisurapanont M, Disayavanish C, Taimkaew K (2000) Quetiapine for Schizophrenia (Cochrane Review). In: *The Cochrane Library,* Issue 3. Oxford: Update Software

Stanniland C, Taylor D (2000) Tolerability of atypical antipsychotics. *Drug Safety* 22, 195–214.

Stephenson C, Bigliani V, Kerwin W et al (2000) The action of quetiapine at striatal and extra-striatal D2/D3 receptors in vivo. *Br J Psychiatry* 177, 408–16.

Stone J, Ohlsen R, Taylor D, Pilowsky LS (2002) A naturalistic study of the antipsychotic medication review service at the Maudsley Hospital. *Psychiatric Bull* (in press).

Taylor D (1997) Pharmacokinetic interactions involving clozapine. *Br J Psychiatry* 171, 109–12.

Taylor D (1997b) Switching from typical to atypical antipsychotics; Practical Guidelines. *CNS Drugs* 8(4), 285–92.

Taylor D (2000) Low dose typical antipsychotics – an evaluation. *Psychiatric Bull* 24, 465–8.

Taylor D, Knapp M, Kerwin RW (2002) Pharmacoeconomics in psychiatry. London: Martin Dunitz Ltd.

Taylor D, McAskill R (2000) Atypical antipsychotics and weight gain – a systematic review. *Acta Psychiatr Scand* 101, 416–32.

Taylor D, Shapland L, Laverick G et al (2000) Clozapine – a survey of patient perceptions. *Psychiatric Bull* 24, 450–52.

Taylor DM (2002) Antipsychotics and QT prolongation. *Acta Psychiatr Scand* (in press).

Travis MJ, Busatto GF, Pilowsky LS et al (1998) 5HT2a receptor blockade in schizophrenic patients treated with risperidone or clozapine, a 123I-5-I-R-91150 single photon emission tomography (SPET) study. *Br J Psychiatry* 173, 236–42.

Trichard C, Paillere-Martinot ML, Attar-Levy D (1998) Binding of antipsychotic drugs to cortical 5-HT2A receptors: a PET study of chlorpromazine, clozapine, and amisulpride in schizophrenic patients. *Am J Psychiatry* 155(4), 505–8.

United States Department of Health, Education and Welfare 1995. Abnormal involuntary movements scale (AIMS). In: Weiner WJ, Lang AE, eds. (1995) *Behavioural Neurology of Mental Disorders; Advances in Neurology.* Vol 65, New York: Raven Press.

Voruganti L, Cortese L, Oyewumi L et al (2000) Comparative evaluation of conventional and novel antipsychotic drugs with reference to their subjective tolerability, side-effect profile and impact on quality of life. *Schizophrenia Res* 43, 135–45.

Wahlbeck K, Cheine M, Essali MA (2000) Clozapine versus typical neuroleptic medication for schizophrenia (Cochrane Review). In: *The Cochrane Library,* Issue 3. Oxford: Update Software.

Wilkinson G, Hedson B, Wild D et al (200) Self-report quality of life measure for people with schizophrenia: The SQLS. *Br J Psychiatry* 177, 42–6.

Wing JK, Beevor AS, Curtis RH (1998) Health of the Nation Outcome Scales (Ho NOS). Research and development. *Br J Psychiatry* 172, 11–18 [Abstract].

Zimbroff DL, Kane JM, Tamminga C et al (1997) Controlled, dose response study of sertindole and haloperidol in the treatment of schizophrenia. *Am J Psychiatry* 154, 782–91.

Index